FIRST AID FAST
for
Babies
and Children

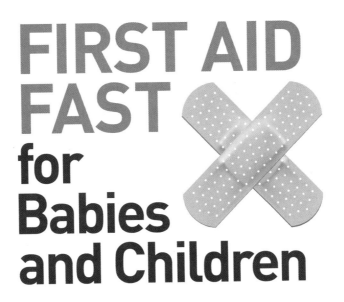

D1341468

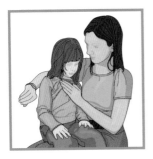
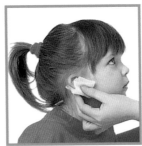
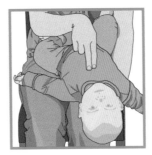
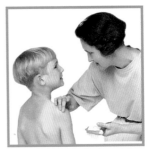

FIRST AID
FAST
for
Babies
and Children

Emergency procedures for all parents and carers

Medical Editor

Dr Vivien J Armstrong

DK

DK LONDON

Consultant Editor Jemima Dunne
Senior Art Editor Sharon Spencer
Project Editor Miezan van Zyl
Jacket Designer Mark Cavanagh
Managing Editor Angeles Gavira
Managing Art Editor Michael Duffy
Pre-Production Producer Andy Hilliard
Producer Jude Crozier
Art Director Karen Self
Associate Publishing Director Liz Wheeler
Publishing Director Jonathan Metcalf

DK INDIA

Art Editors Konica Juneja, Anjali Sachar
Senior DTP Designers Harish Aggarwal, Vishal Bhatia
Managing Editor Rohan Sinha
Deputy Managing Art Editor Anjana Nair
Pre-production Manager Balwant Singh
Production Manager Pankaj Sharma
Jacket Designer Dhirendra Singh
Editorial coordinator Priyanka Sharma
Managing Jackets Editor Sreshtha Bhattacharya

First published in Great Britain as *First Aid for Children Fast* in 1994;
revised in 1999, 2002, 2006, 2012, 2017
This sixth edition published 2017 by Dorling Kindersley Limited,
80 Strand, London WC2R 0RL

A CIP catalogue record for this book is available from the British Library
ISBN 978-0-2411-9873-5

Printed and bound in China

A WORLD OF IDEAS:
SEE ALL THERE IS TO KNOW

www.dk.com

Disclaimer:
First Aid Fast for Babies and Children provides information and guidance on initial care following an incident or if
a child is unwell, but should not be regarded as a substitute for medical advice. The publisher and medical editor
do not accept responsibility for any claims arising from the use of this manual.

Foreword

Would you know what to do if your child fell over and cut his arm or tripped and injured his ankle? Would you have the confidence to manage the injury, comfort your child, and know where to get help? Could you look after your baby who has a raised temperature and be able to recognise when an illness becomes more serious?

Children are naturally adventurous and suffering minor injuries is all part of growing up, as are childhood illnesses, and fortunately serious injuries and illnesses are rare. Whatever the incident though, it is important that a child receives the best possible first aid at the time. Good initial care can not only preserve life, but is also likely to improve the recovery process. This revised edition of *First Aid Fast for Babies and Children* contains all of the latest guidelines for saving life as well as guidance on how to deal with less serious injuries and illnesses.

I hope the advice and guidance in this book will provide you with the knowledge, skills, and confidence to look after any child or baby who has an injury or illness and also help you to feel confident to take action if a serious incident occurs.

Dr Vivien J Armstrong MBBS FRCA DRCOG PGCE (FE)
Medical Editor

Contents

Introduction 8

How to use this book 9

Action in an
Emergency 10
Fire 11
Electrical injury 12
Water incident 13
Checking vital signs 14

Unresponsiveness 16
Unresponsiveness 16
Unresponsive baby 19
CPR: baby 20
Unresponsive child 22
CPR: child 24
Recovery position 26

Breathing Difficulties 28
Choking baby 28
Choking child 30
Breath holding 32
Hiccups 32

Suffocation and
strangulation 33
Fume inhalation 33
Croup 34
Asthma 35

Wounds and Bleeding 36
Shock 36
Severe bleeding 38
Embedded object 40
Cuts and grazes 41
Infected wound 42
Blisters 43
Eye wound 44
Nosebleed 45
Ear wound 46
Mouth wound 47
Amputation 48
Internal bleeding 49

Crush injury 49
Chest wound 50
Abdominal wound 51

Burns and Scalds 52
Burns and scalds 52
Electrical burn 54
Chemical burn to skin 55
Chemical burn to eye 56

Poisoning 57
Swallowed chemicals 57
Drug and alcohol poisoning 58
Plant poisoning 58

Head, Face, and
Spine Injuries 59
Scalp wound 59
Head injury 60
Nose/cheekbone injury 62
Jaw injury 62
Spine injury 63

Bone, Joint, and
Muscle Injuries 64
Pelvic injury 64
Leg injury 64
Knee injury 66
Foot injury 66
Ankle injury 67
Collar bone injury 68
Rib injury 69
Arm injury 70
Elbow injury 70

Hand injury 71
Finger injury 72
Cramp 73
Bruises and swellings 74

Foreign Objects 75
Splinter 75
Object in eye 76
Object in ear 77
Object in nose 78
Swallowed object 78

Bites and Stings 79
Animal and human bites 79
Insect sting 80
Nettle rash 80
Tick bite 81
Jellyfish sting 82
Marine puncture wound 82
Snake bite 83

Effects of Heat and Cold 84
Hypothermia 84
Frostbite 86
Sunburn 87
Heat rash 87
Heat exhaustion 88
Heatstroke 89

Medical Disorders 90
Allergy 90
Anaphylactic shock 91

Diabetic emergency 92
Faint 93
Fever 94
Meningitis 95
Febrile seizures 96
Epileptic seizures 97
Vomiting and diarrhoea 98
Stomachache 99
Earache 100
Toothache 101

First Aid Kit 102
First aid kit 102
Dressings 104
Bandaging 105
Triangular bandages 106
Useful household items 108

Home Safety 109
Safety at home 109
Hall and stairs 110
Sitting room 111
Kitchen 112
Bedrooms 114
Bathroom 116
Toys and playthings 117
Garden 118

Garage and car safety 119
Out and about 120
Travelling with children 122

Index 123
Acknowledgments 127

Useful Telephone Numbers 128

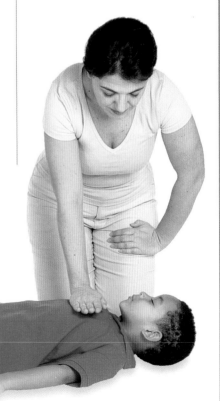

Introduction

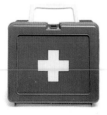 This book has been compiled primarily for parents but also for others – grandparents, teachers, childminders, playgroup leaders, and babysitters – who may regularly, or even occasionally, find themselves in charge of babies and children. The content has been set out in a clear and logical way and the information presented largely in pictorial form using simple words and captions to make it very easy to follow and to understand. The first aid advice given can be used to treat any age child up to puberty and follows the most up-to-date clinical guidance at the time of publication.

Emergencies are, by their very nature, unexpected events and can be extremely frightening and stressful for anyone caring for a child. *First Aid Fast for Babies and Children* will help you to learn various practical skills that will help you to cope with a range of first aid emergencies and everyday accidents, building your confidence and ensuring that you respond in the best way possible. The calmer you are the more effective your help will be, and by listening and talking to the child you will be able to make the best decision for both you and him or her, greatly improving the outcome.

In addition there is reference information at the back of the book. A section on first aid kits and bandaging techniques also lists useful items to have at home and how to use them. The pages on Home Safety highlight potential danger areas around the home and how to fix them to minimise the risk of incidents in the first place.

How to use this book

This book covers first aid treatment for everything from minor cuts and grazes to treating a child who is not responding. For every condition a series of photographs or artworks shows you exactly what to do in an emergency. Key pieces of information are indicated on the photographs and supplementary advice can be found alongside in the step-by-step text.

The injuries are organised by type, in coloured sections such as Breathing Difficulties or Wounds and Bleeding. However, in an emergency, the thumbnail index on the back cover will direct you straight to the relevant page. There are also sections, such as Action in an Emergency, Bandages and Dressings, and Home Safety, that contain information for general reference.

Key signs and symptoms help you to recognise the conditions

Annotations highlight essential action

Clear photographs illustrate every step of treatment

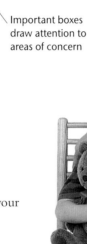

Important boxes draw attention to areas of concern

Symbols highlight the action necessary for medical help

Cross-references direct you to pages with information about associated injuries

Guide to the symbols

The following symbols and instructions appear if your child needs further medical attention:

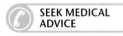 **SEEK MEDICAL ADVICE**

Depending on your area, call your doctor's surgery, nurse practitioner, on-call service, or NHS 111 for advice.

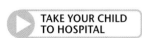 **TAKE YOUR CHILD TO HOSPITAL**

Take your child to the nearest hospital accident and emergency department if you have help and transport.

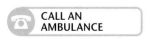 **CALL AN AMBULANCE**

Your child needs urgent medical attention and is best transported by ambulance to hospital.

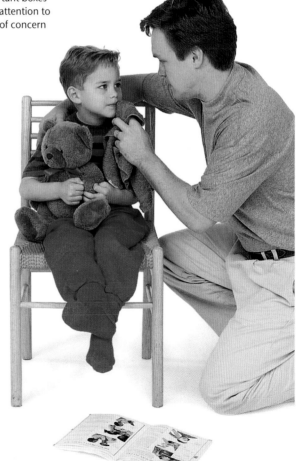

Action in an emergency

In any emergency, particularly one involving children, it is important to keep calm and act logically. Remember four steps:

 ## Assess the situation

- What happened and how did it happen?
- Is it safe for you to approach?
- Is there more than one injured child?
- Is there anyone who can help?
- Do you need the emergency services?

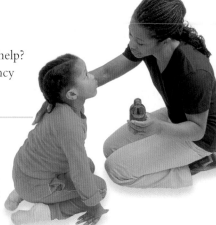

 ## Safety is important

- Do not risk injuring yourself – you cannot help if you become a casualty.
- Remove any source of danger from your child. Move your child only if it is safe for you and it's essential for her safety, and do it very carefully.

 ## Treat serious injuries first

The primary considerations that immediately threaten life are:
- Obstructed airway, which prevents breathing, for example as a result of unresponsiveness (*see p. 14*).
- Serious bleeding, which can result in life-threatening shock (*see p. 36*).

> **! IMPORTANT**
>
> - **If** more than one child is injured go to the quiet one – she may be unresponsive and not breathing.

Get help

Shout for help early and ask others to:
- Make the area safe.
- Seek medical advice or call an ambulance.
- Help with first aid.
- Move a child to safety, if necessary.

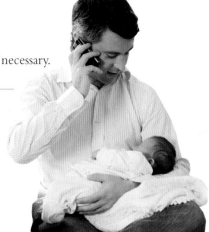

Telephoning for help

When you call the emergency services use the hands-free facility so you can treat the child while you make the call. Provide the following:
- Your telephone number.
- The location of the incident.
- The type of incident.
- The number, sex, and ages of the casualties.
- Details of injuries.
- Information about hazards such as gas, power lines, or fog.

Fire

Write down an escape plan for your home and make sure everyone knows what to do.
- How would you get out of each room?
- How do you help babies and young children?
- Where will you meet when you've escaped?

Action for a chip pan fire

- Turn off heat source, then cover pan with lid, wet tea towel, or fire blanket – leave this on for half an hour – NEVER throw water over the flames.
- If fire is not under control, get out of the house, closing doors behind you, and call the fire brigade.

Escaping from a fire

1 Feel the door. If the door is cool, leave the room.

OR

2 If the door is hot, don't open it. Go to the window.

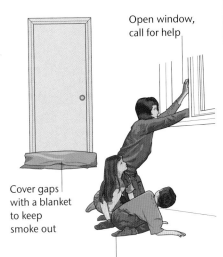

Shut the door behind you

Leave quickly
DO NOT GO BACK

Open window, call for help

Cover gaps with a blanket to keep smoke out

Stay low down where air is clearest

! IMPORTANT

- **Carry** babies and toddlers.
- **Don't** ask children to do anything other than look after themselves.
- **Close** all doors behind you.
- **Meet** outside your house.
- **Never** go back inside.
- **Phone** for help from elsewhere.

If you have to escape through a window:
- **If** you have to break the glass, put a blanket over the frame before you escape.
- **Slide** your child out, hang onto him, then ask him to drop down.
- **Slide** out yourself, hang from the ledge, then drop.

Clothing on fire

If clothing is on fire:
Stop your child moving as movement will fan the flames.
Drop him to the floor and wrap him in a coat or blanket to help smother the flames.
Roll him on the ground.

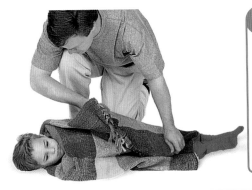

! IMPORTANT

- **Do not** let your child run about in a panic; rapid movement will fan the flames.

- **If** water is available, lay him down, burning side uppermost, and douse him with water or a non-flammable liquid.

! IMPORTANT

● **Never** touch your child's skin. Pull at his clothes as a last resort.

● **If** your child is no longer in contact with the electricity and is unresponsive, open his airway and check breathing. If breathing, place in the recovery position; if not breathing, begin CPR immediately. CALL AN AMBULANCE

High-voltage current

Contact with electricity from power lines and overhead cables is usually fatal. Severe burns result and the child may be thrown some distance from the point of contact. DO NOT approach the child unless you are officially informed that the power has been cut off.

» see also

● Checking vital signs, p.14

● Electrical burns, p.54

● Unresponsive baby, pp.19–21

● Unresponsive child, pp.22–27

Electrical injury

Children are at risk of injury from domestic electricity if they play with electrical sockets or flexes, or if flexes are worn. Electrical current causes muscle spasms that prevent a child letting go of an electric cable and may cause burns both where the current enters and leaves the child's body. The current may also cause breathing and heart to stop.

☎ CALL AN AMBULANCE

1 Do not touch the child. Break the contact with electricity by switching the current off at the mains.

2 If you cannot switch off the current, stand on dry insulating material such as telephone books or a wooden box. Use a wooden broom handle or chair to separate your child's limbs from the source.

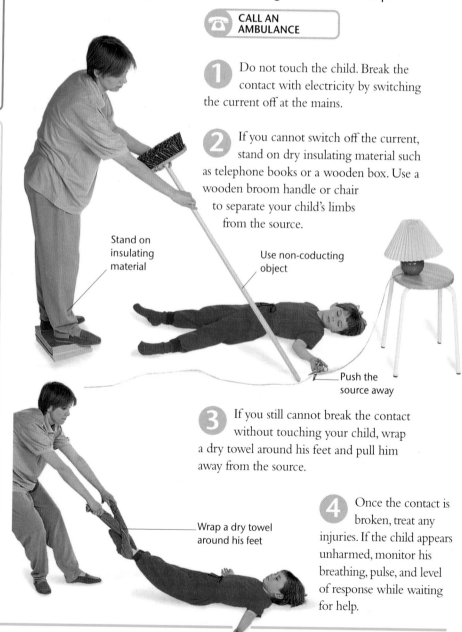

Stand on insulating material

Use non-coducting object

Push the source away

3 If you still cannot break the contact without touching your child, wrap a dry towel around his feet and pull him away from the source.

Wrap a dry towel around his feet

4 Once the contact is broken, treat any injuries. If the child appears unharmed, monitor his breathing, pulse, and level of response while waiting for help.

Water incident

Babies and young children can drown quickly if they slip into a pool or pond or are left unattended in a bath. Even 2.5cm (1in) of water is enough to cover a baby's nose and mouth if he falls forwards.

! **IMPORTANT**

● **Do not** put yourself in danger when attempting a rescue; don't enter the water unless you are a trained lifesaver.

● **If** you are a trained lifesaver and the child is unresponsive wade into the water to rescue him. Tow him ashore keeping him as upright as possible.

● **Always** seek medical advice even if the child appears to have recovered as he may have inhaled some water, which can cause lung damage.

● **If** the child becomes unresponsive, open his airway and check breathing. If breathing, place in the recovery position; if not breathing, begin CPR immediately. CALL AN AMBULANCE.

● **Be** prepared to roll child onto his side to clear airway because he is likely to regurgitate his stomach contents.

1 Get the child out of the water as quickly as possible. Stay on the bank and hold out a branch or rope for the child to grab, or throw him a float. Lie on the bank or get someone else to hold you as you lean out to the child.

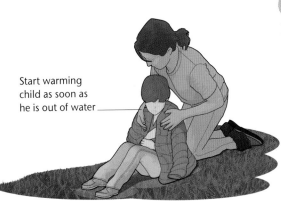

Hold a sturdy branch and tell child to grab it

Lie on bank so you don't fall in

2 Once the child is out of the water protect him from cold and get him to a shelter. Treat him for hypothermia and replace any wet clothes with dry ones as soon as possible. Even if the child seems to have recovered,

Start warming child as soon as he is out of water

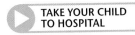
▶ TAKE YOUR CHILD TO HOSPITAL

OR

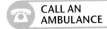
☎ CALL AN AMBULANCE

DROWNING CHAIN OF SURVIVAL

Prevent drowning	Recognize distress	Provide flotation	Remove from water	Give first aid
Stay safe and supervise your child in and around water.	Ask someone to call for help if a person is in distress.	Getting a float to a child can prevent submersion.	Only attempt this if it is safe to do so.	Treat as appropriate and seek medical advice.

» *see also*

● Hypothermia, *p.84*

● Unresponsive baby, *pp.19–21*

● Unresponsive child, *pp.22–27*

Checking vital signs

When you are looking after a baby or child who is ill or injured you need to check her vital signs – breathing, pulse, and level of response – as part of assessing the severity of a condition. Then continue to monitor all three signs while you are looking after your child or waiting for medical help to arrive, as the information can indicate whether a child's condition is changing (either improving or deteriorating). Note that here you are checking and monitoring for quality of pulse or breathing, not presence or absence of them.

Breathing

When assessing breathing, you are looking at how many times a child breathes in a minute, as well as the quality of the breaths – for example depth and ease. An older child breathes about 12–16 breaths a minute; a baby or young child can breathe as much as 35 times.

You can sit with the child and watch and listen for breaths, or for a baby or younger child it may be better to place your hand on the chest. Make a note of the breathing rate (the number of breaths in a minute) and as well as whether they are deep or shallow, easy or difficult, painful and/or quiet or noisy – and if the latter, what do they sound like?

Time the breaths with your watch

Check breathing Rate
Sit your child down or on your lap. Place one hand on her chest. Count the number of times she breathes in a minute and listen to the breaths.

Pulse

Every time the heart beats, a wave of pressure passes along the blood vessels that carry blood from the heart to the body (arteries). This "wave" can be felt where the arteries lie close to the skin. For a baby, check the pulse in the upper arm, for older children check it at the wrist. The normal pulse rate for an older child is 60–80 beats per minute and it can be up to 160 beats in young children. Count the rate (number of beats in a minute), and note whether it is strong or weak and regular or irregular.

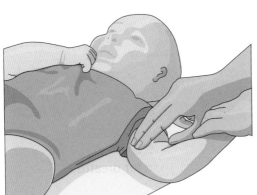

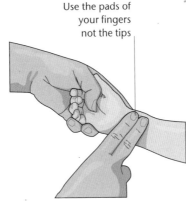

Use the pads of
your fingers
not the tips

BRACHIAL PULSE

Place the pads of two fingers (not your fingertips as they have a pulse of their own) against the inner side of the baby's upper arm.

RADIAL PULSE

Place the pads of two or three fingers on the forearm just below the wrist creases at the base of the thumb.

Level of response

Some illnesses and injuries can affect your child's level of response and she may be fully alert or totally unresponsive or somewhere inbetween. Assess your child straightaway and then again at regular intervals.

- *Child is fully alert* Her eyes will be open and she responds normally when you ask questions.
- *Responds only to voice* Does your child answer simple questions and obey instructions? Can she open her eyes?
- *Responds only to pain* Does your child open her eyes or move if you tap her shoulder or flick her foot?
- *Unresponsive* The child does not respond to any stimulus.

Body temperature

This is not strictly speaking a vital sign, but a temperature above or below normal can be a sign of illness.

- A body temperature above 37°C (98.6) is a sign of a fever – a moderate fever is not harmful, but above 39°C (102.2°F) it is potentially serious. A body temperature below 35°C (95°F) indicates hypothermia.

- Don't put a digital thermometer in a young child's mouth. Place it in the armpit instead and lower the arm over it. The temperature recorded will be 0.5°C (1°F) degree lower – so a reading of 36.5°C (97.6°F) is a fever.

Unresponsiveness

A baby or child needs to inhale oxygen into his lungs. This oxygen passes into the bloodstream and is pumped around the body by the heart. If a baby or child is unresponsive, the air passage, or airway, to the lungs may be blocked, which means oxygen can't enter the body. Lack of oxygen slows down the heartbeat until it stops altogether (cardiac arrest) and no oxygen will reach the brain.

What you can do to help

Always make sure it is safe to approach the baby or child; you can't help him if you become a casualty too. If you are certain you are safe, first assess whether he is responsive. If he is unresponsive, you must open the airway and check breathing. Then, if necessary, breathe into his lungs – this is known as rescue breathing. If circulation stops, blood cannot travel around the body and vital organs such as the brain and heart are deprived of oxygen so you need to help to pump some blood by doing chest compressions. The combination of rescue breaths and chest compressions is known as cardiopulmonary resuscitation (CPR). An AED can be used to restore a normal heartbeat in a child over the age of one (see *p.23*).

Chain of survival

An unresponsive baby or child's chances of survival are greater if:

- You call for expert help;
- CPR is given as soon as possible;
- An AED is used early (on a child only);
- Advanced care by healthcare professionals is received as soon as possible.

For a baby Call his name and tap foot to check for response

For a child

Call your child's name and tap shoulder to check for a response

Open the airway

You need to open the airway before you can check breathing. Place one hand on the forehead and gently tilt the head to bring the tongue away from the back of the throat. Place one or two fingers of your other hand on the chin to lift. If you suspect a neck injury, use the jaw thrust method to open the airway (see *p.61*).

Airway

If child is on his back the tongue falls back and blocks the airway.

Tongue fallen back

Head not tilted – airway blocked

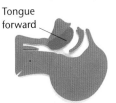

Tongue forward

Head tilted – airway unblocked

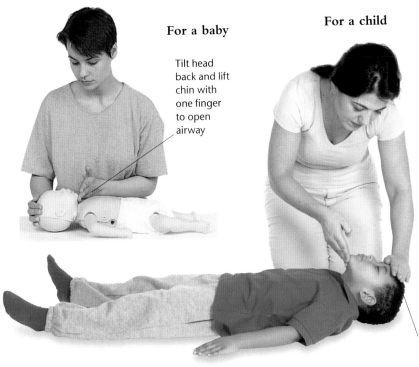

For a baby

Tilt head back and lift chin with one finger to open airway

For a child

Tilt head back and lift chin with two fingers to open airway

Breathe for the baby or child

If your baby or child is not breathing after the airway has been opened, take a breath and blow oxygen into the child's lungs. This is known as rescue breathing.

For a child

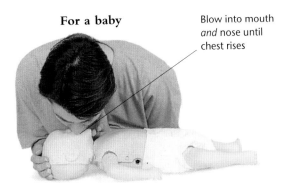

For a baby

Blow into mouth *and* nose until chest rises

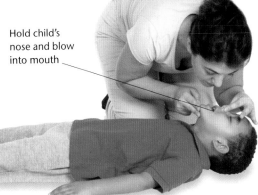

Hold child's nose and blow into mouth

Maintain blood circulation

If your baby or child's heart has stopped beating, giving chest compressions will drive blood containing oxygen around the body. These will be more effective if alternated with rescue breaths. The combination of techniques is known as cardiopulmonary resuscitation (CPR).

For a baby

For a child

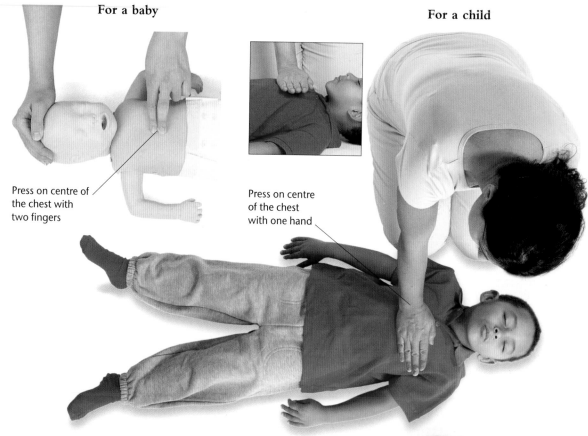

Press on centre of the chest with two fingers

Press on centre of the chest with one hand

When to call an ambulance

If there is somebody else present to help, always ask him or her to call an ambulance as soon as you realise that your child is not breathing. If you are on your own, give a combination of rescue breaths and chest compressions (CPR: baby *p.20*, child *p.24*) for one minute before stopping to make the call. Then continue CPR until help arrives or the child recovers.

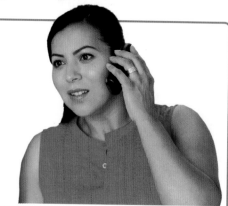

Unresponsive baby

Assess your baby before calling for help. If you are alone and the baby is not breathing, begin rescue breaths and chest compressions.

① Check for response

- Call her name and tap her foot gently. Never shake a baby.
- If there is no response, continue to step 2.
- If there is a response,

 SEEK MEDICAL ADVICE

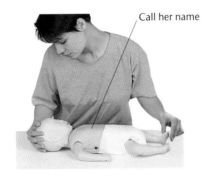

Call her name

② Open baby's airway

- Put one hand on the baby's forehead and gently tilt her head.
- Place one finger of your other hand on the tip of her chin and lift it.

! IMPORTANT
- **Do not** press the soft part of the neck under the chin as it can block the airway.

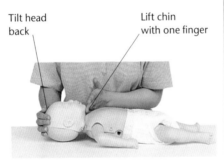

Tilt head back

Lift chin with one finger

③ Check breathing for no more than 10 seconds

- Look, listen, and feel for breathing. Look along her chest for movement, listen for sounds of breathing, and feel for breaths against your cheek. Send helper to:

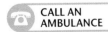 **CALL AN AMBULANCE**

- If she is breathing, cradle her in your arms with head tilted down and wait for help.
- If she is not breathing begin CPR – GO TO PAGE 20.

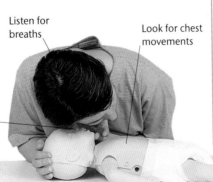

Listen for breaths

Look for chest movements

Feel for breath on your cheek

Resuscitation summary

Unconscious baby

Airway open

No breathing

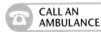

Send helper to

 CALL AN AMBULANCE

Begin CPR: give five initial rescue breaths, followed by 30 compressions then two rescue breaths.

Repeat 30:2 for one minute

If not already done,

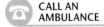 **CALL AN AMBULANCE**

Continue CPR until help arrives

! IMPORTANT
- **If** you are unable or unwilling to give rescue breaths you can give chest compressions only.

Resuscitation summary

Unresponsive baby

Airway open

No breathing

Send helper to

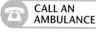
CALL AN AMBULANCE

Begin CPR: give five initial rescue breaths, followed by 30 chest compressions then two rescue breaths

Repeat 30:2 for one minute

If not already done,

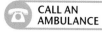
CALL AN AMBULANCE

Continue CPR until help arrives

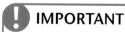
! IMPORTANT

• If you are unable or unwilling to give rescue breaths you can give chest compressions only.

CPR: baby

This is to be used for an unresponsive baby who is not breathing. Always give five initial rescue breaths before beginning chest compressions. If on your own, give CPR for one minute before calling an ambulance.

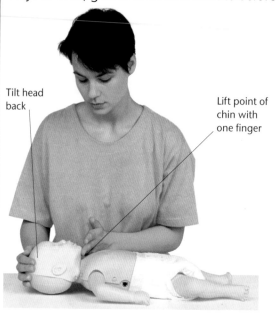

Tilt head back

Lift point of chin with one finger

1 Make sure that her airway is open. Put your fingers on the point of the chin and lift it. Take care not to press on the soft part of the neck under the chin as that can block the airway.

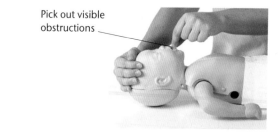

Pick out visible obstructions

2 Pick out any visible obstruction from the mouth and nose with your fingertips.

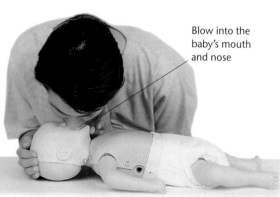

Blow into the baby's mouth and nose

3 Take a normal breath, then seal your lips tightly around your baby's mouth and nose. Blow gently until you see the baby's chest rise.

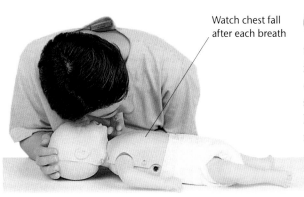

Watch chest fall
after each breath

4 Remove your mouth and watch the chest fall back – this is a rescue breath. Each complete rescue breath should take one second. Repeat to give five rescue breaths.

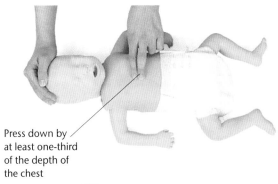

Press down by
at least one-third
of the depth of
the chest

5 Begin chest compressions. Place two fingers of your lower hand on the centre of the baby's chest. Press down vertically on the breastbone to depress it by at least one third of its depth. Release pressure, but don't move your fingers; allow the chest to come back up fully. Repeat to give 30 compressions at a rate of 100–120 per minute.

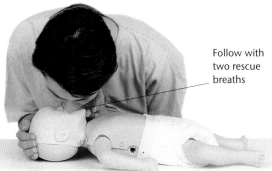

Follow with
two rescue
breaths

6 Return to the baby's head and give TWO rescue breaths this time, followed by another 30 chest compressions. Continue at a rate of 30:2 until the emergency services arrive; your baby shows signs of becoming responsive (coughing, opening her eyes, and moving purposefully) and she is breathing normally; or you are too exhausted to continue.

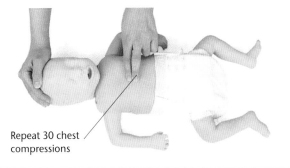

Repeat 30 chest
compressions

IMPORTANT

- **Do not** sweep the mouth with your finger to search for an obstruction.

- **Make** up to five attempts at rescue breaths before beginning chest compressions.

- **If** there is more than one rescuer swap every two minutes with minimal interruption to compressions.

- **If** your baby shows signs of becoming responsive (*see left*) and she is breathing normally, cradle her in your arms with head tilted down until the ambulance arrives (*below*). Monitor breathing, pulse, and level of response (*p.14*) until the help arrives.

The recovery position

Hold the baby in your arms with her head tilted downwards and supported. This keeps her airway open and clear and allows fluid to drain away.

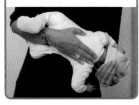

Resuscitation summary

Unresponsive child

⬇

Airway open

⬇

No breathing

⬇

Send helper to

 CALL AN AMBULANCE

⬇

Begin CPR: give five initial rescue breaths, followed by 30 chest compressions then two rescue breaths

⬇

Repeat 30:2 for one minute

⬇

If not already done,

 CALL AN AMBULANCE

⬇

Continue CPR until help arrives

! IMPORTANT
● If you are unable or unwilling to give rescue breaths you can give chest compressions only.

Unresponsive child

Assess a child (aged one year to puberty) before you call for help. If you are on your own and the child is not breathing, begin CPR.

① Check for response

● Call his name, or tap his shoulder gently. Never shake a child.
● If there is no response, go to step 2.
● If there is a response,

 SEEK MEDICAL ADVICE

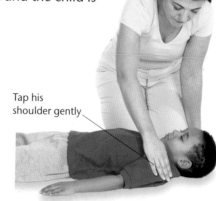

Tap his shoulder gently

② Open child's airway

● Put one hand on the child's forehead and gently tilt his head back.
● Place two fingers of your other hand on the tip of his chin and lift it.

! IMPORTANT
● **Do not** press the soft part of the neck under the chin as it can block the airway.

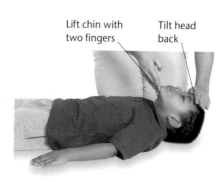

Lift chin with two fingers

Tilt head back

③ Check breathing for no more than 10 seconds

● Look, listen, and feel for breathing. Look along his chest for movement, listen for sounds of breathing, and feel for breaths against your cheek. Send a helper to:

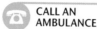 CALL AN AMBULANCE

● If he is breathing place him in the recovery position. GO TO PAGE 26.
● If he not breathing, begin CPR. GO TO PAGE 24.

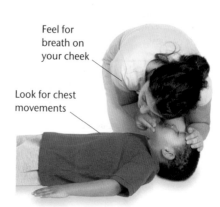

Feel for breath on your cheek

Look for chest movements

Using an AED on a child

Machines called AEDs can be used to analyse the heart rhythm and if necessary correct it by delivering an electric shock. If a child is unresponsive and not breathing, start rescue breaths and chest compressions (CPR, *see p.24*), CALL AN AMBULANCE. Ask a helper to find an AED and use it as soon as it arrives – don't leave the child to look for one yourself. The machine will give you a series of audible prompts to follow. If a shock is needed the machine will deliver it; if it is not needed it also knows not to deliver one.

1 Put the AED beside the child, open the lid and take out the electrode pads – they will be attached to the machine.

2 Place the pads directly onto the child's chest. Peel off the backing paper and put one on the upper right side of the child's chest and the other on her lower left side.

3 Once the pads are attached, make sure no-one is touching the child. The AED will analyse the heart rhythm and may recommend delivering a shock. Listen to the machine's instructions.

IF A SHOCK IS ADVISED
● The AED will start to charge up – make sure everyone is clear of the child, then follow the machine's prompts to deliver the shock.
● Continue CPR until the machine asks you to stop.
● The AED will re-analyse the child's heart rhythm at regular intervals; listen to the prompts.

IF A SHOCK IS NOT ADVISED
● Continue CPR. The AED will re-analyse the child's heart rhythm at regular intervals.

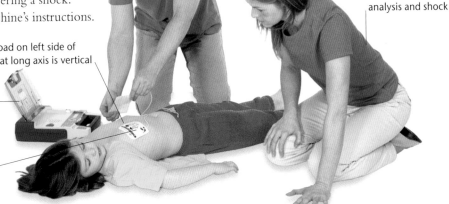

Ask all helpers to stay clear of the child during analysis and shock

Place one pad on left side of chest so that long axis is vertical

AED

Place one pad on upper right side of chest

 IMPORTANT

● **If** a child's (paediatric) AED is not available, you can use an adult machine for a child aged 1–8. Ideally use paediatric pads.

● **Do not** use an AED on a baby under the age of one year.

● **If** the child is very small, place one pad in the centre of her back and the other one in the centre of the chest. Both pads should be vertical.

● **If** she starts coughing, opening her eyes, speaking or moving purposefully, and is breathing normally, leave pads attached and put her in the recovery position.

Resuscitation summary

Unresponsive child

Airway open

No breathing

Send helper to

 CALL AN AMBULANCE

Begin CPR: give five initial rescue breaths, followed by 30 chest compressions then two rescue breaths

Repeat 30:2 for one minute

If not already done,

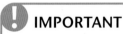 **CALL AN AMBULANCE**

Continue CPR until help arrives

> **⚠ IMPORTANT**
> ● **If** you are unable or unwilling to give rescue breaths you can give chest compressions only.

CPR: child

This is to be used for an unresponsive child who is not breathing. Always give five initial rescue breaths before beginning chest compressions. If on your own, give CPR for one minute before calling an ambulance.

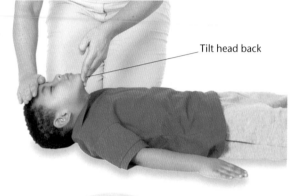

Tilt head back

1 Make sure that the child's airway is open. Put your fingers on the point of the chin and lift it. Take care not to press on the soft part of the neck under the chin, as that can block the airway. Pick out any visible obstructions from the child's mouth with your fingertips.

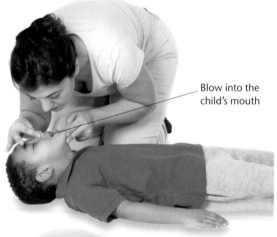

Blow into the child's mouth

2 Pinch the child's nose. Take a normal breath, seal your lips around his mouth and blow steadily into the mouth; the chest should rise.

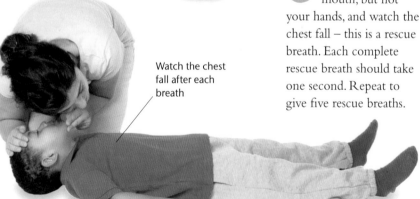

Watch the chest fall after each breath

3 Remove your mouth, but not your hands, and watch the chest fall – this is a rescue breath. Each complete rescue breath should take one second. Repeat to give five rescue breaths.

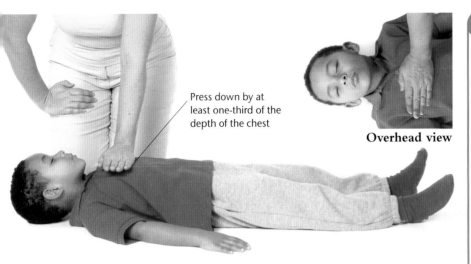

Press down by at least one-third of the depth of the chest

Overhead view

4 Begin chest compressions. Place the heel of one hand over the centre of the child's chest (on the breastbone). Lean forwards over the child so that your shoulder is directly above your hand. Press down vertically to depress the breastbone by at least one third of its depth.

5 Release the pressure but don't move your hand; let the chest come back up. Repeat to give 30 compressions at a rate of 100–120 per minute.

6 Return to the child's head and give two rescue breaths. followed by 30 chest compressions.

7 Continue at a rate of 30:2 until the emergency services arrive; your child shows signs of becoming responsive (coughing, opening eyes, speaking, and moving purposefully) and is breathing normally; or you are too exhausted to continue.

For a larger child or small rescuer

If the child is large, or you are small, you can deliver chest compressions with two hands. Place one hand on the centre of the child's chest, then put your other hand on top and interlock your fingers. Then press down firmly to deliver compressions as above.

Interlock your fingers

Keep your fingers off the child's chest

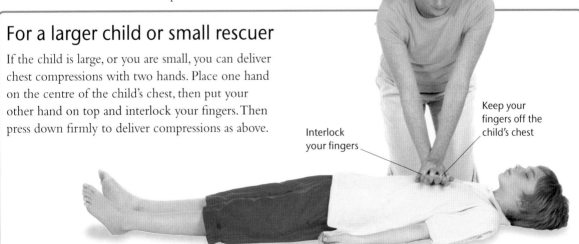

Spectacles

If the child is wearing spectacles, remove them and keep them safe.

Recovery position

Put your child in this position if she is unresponsive but breathing to prevent her tongue or vomit from blocking her airway. If the child is found lying on her side or front not all the steps will be needed.

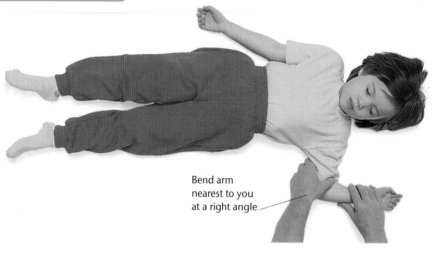

1 Kneel beside your child. Place the arm closest to you up alongside her head with the elbow bent and palm of hand uppermost.

Bend arm nearest to you at a right angle

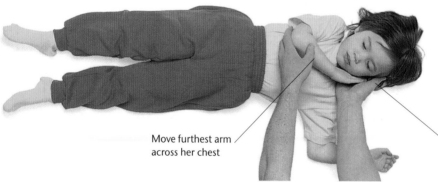

2 Bring her other arm across her chest and hold the back of her hand against her cheek.

Move furthest arm across her chest

Hold hand against her cheek

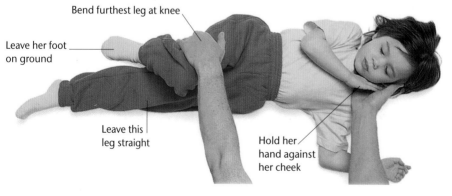

Bend furthest leg at knee

Leave her foot on ground

Leave this leg straight

Hold her hand against her cheek

3 With your other hand, pull up the knee of the leg furthest away from you to bend the leg, leaving the foot on the ground.

4 Pull the bent leg towards you to roll your child onto her side. Keep your child's hand against her cheek to support her head.

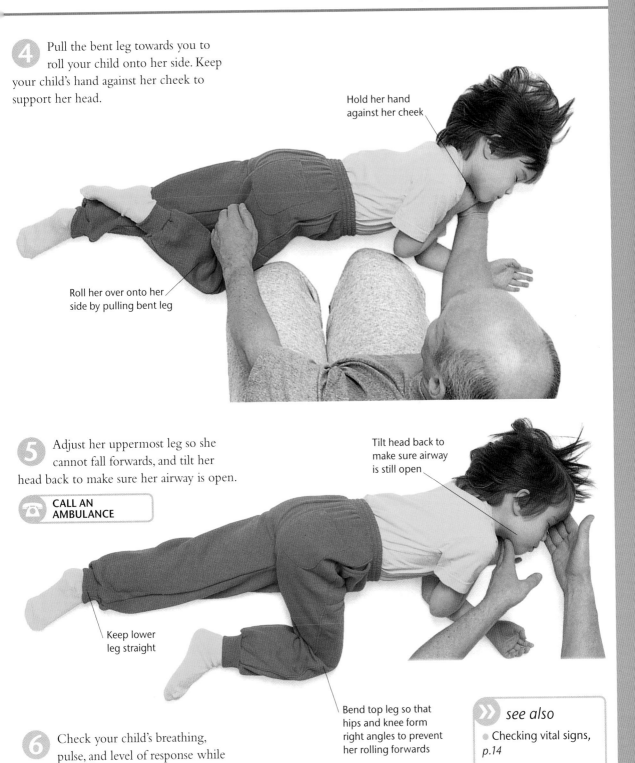

Hold her hand against her cheek

Roll her over onto her side by pulling bent leg

5 Adjust her uppermost leg so she cannot fall forwards, and tilt her head back to make sure her airway is open.

📞 **CALL AN AMBULANCE**

Tilt head back to make sure airway is still open

Keep lower leg straight

6 Check your child's breathing, pulse, and level of response while you are waiting for help to arrive.

Bend top leg so that hips and knee form right angles to prevent her rolling forwards

》 see also
● Checking vital signs, *p.14*

Choking baby

If the choking is mild, your baby will still be able to cough, cry and breathe. If the blockage is severe, however, he will be unable to cough, cry, or breathe. Give back blows then chest thrusts to relieve a blockage.

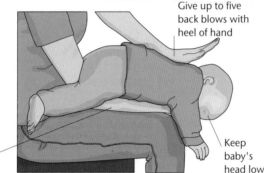

Give up to five back blows with heel of hand

Rest your forearm on your thigh for additional support

Keep baby's head low

1 If your baby is unable to cough, cry, or breathe, lay him face down, head lower than his bottom, along your forearm and rest your arm on your thigh. Support the baby's head with your hand. Give up to five back blows between his shoulder blades with the heel of your other hand.

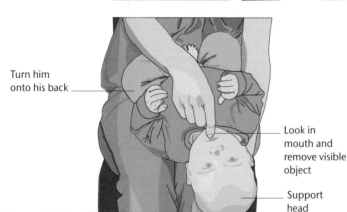

Turn him onto his back

Look in mouth and remove visible object

Support head

2 Turn him face up along your other arm. Check the mouth. Pick out any obvious obstruction from the mouth or nose with your fingertips.

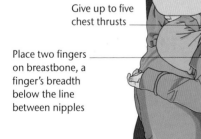

Give up to five chest thrusts

Place two fingers on breastbone, a finger's breadth below the line between nipples

3 If the obstruction has not cleared, give chest thrusts. Place two fingers on the lower half of the baby's breastbone (one finger's breadth below the nipple line) and push downwards. Repeat to give up to five thrusts; stop if the obstruction clears. Check his mouth again. If the obstruction has still not cleared,

☎ **CALL AN AMBULANCE**

4 Continue back blows (step 1 and 3) followed by chest thrusts until help arrives, the obstruction clears, or the baby becomes unresponsive.

If your baby becomes unresponsive

If your choking baby becomes unresponsive, begin CPR. If he starts breathing at any stage, cradle him in your arms with his head down in the recovery position (*see p.21*).

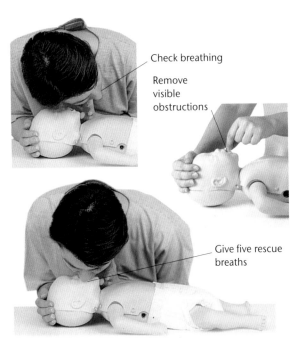

Check breathing

Remove visible obstructions

Give five rescue breaths

Give 30 chest compressions

Place two fingers on the centre of of the chest

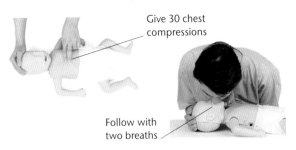

Give 30 chest compressions

Follow with two breaths

1 Open the airway and look, listen, and feel for breathing.

2 If your baby is not breathing, clear any visible obstruction from his mouth and nose; do not do a fingersweep.

3 Begin rescue breaths. Give FIVE initial rescue breaths by breathing into your baby's mouth and nose.

4 Give 30 chest compressions (this may dislodge obstruction), then repeat TWO rescue breaths. Continue to give 30 compressions followed by two rescue breaths for one minute.

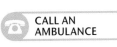 **CALL AN AMBULANCE**

5 Continue alternating 30 chest compressions with two rescue breaths until help arrives, your baby shows signs of recovery (*see box, right*), or you are too exhausted to continue.

! **IMPORTANT**

● **If your baby shows signs of recovery** such as coughing, opening his eyes, and moving purposefully and is breathing normally, CALL AN AMBULANCE if not already done. Cradle him in your arms with head tilted down (recovery position) until the ambulance arrives. Monitor breathing, pulse, and level of response until the ambulance arrives.

» *see also*

● Checking vital signs. *p.14*

● Unresponsive baby, *pp.19–21*

Choking child

Start by asking your child if he is choking. If the blockage is mild, he will be able to speak, cough, and breathe. If it is severe, he will not be able to speak, cough, or breathe.

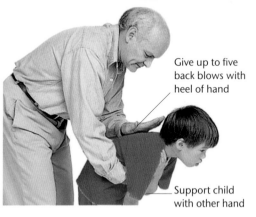

Give up to five back blows with heel of hand

Support child with other hand

1 If your child can cough, encourage him to do so to remove the object.

2 If your child cannot talk, cough, or breathe, help him to bend forwards. Give him up to five back blows between the shoulder blades with the heel of your hand. Check his mouth. Remove any object you can see.

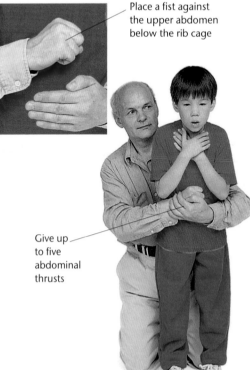

Place a fist against the upper abdomen below the rib cage

Give up to five abdominal thrusts

3 If the obstruction has not cleared, give abdominal thrusts. Place your fist in the middle of his upper abdomen, just below his rib cage. Cover the fist with your other hand and pull sharply inwards and upwards. Repeat to give up to five thrusts; stop if obstruction clears.

4 Check his mouth again. If the obstruction has still not cleared,

☎ **CALL AN AMBULANCE**

5 Continue back blows followed by abdominal thrusts (step 2 and 3) until help arrives, the obstruction clears, or the child becomes unresponsive.

If your child becomes unresponsive

If your choking child becomes unresponsive treat as here. If he starts breathing at any stage, place him in the recovery position and monitor him until help arrives.

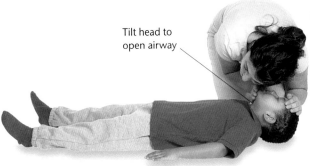

Tilt head to open airway

1 Open his airway. Look, listen, and feel for breathing. If your child is not breathing, pick out any visible obstruction from his mouth; do not do a finger sweep.

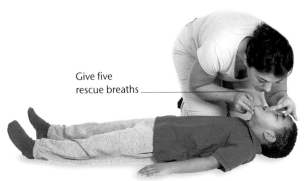

Give five rescue breaths

2 Begin rescue breaths. Give FIVE initial rescue breaths.

3 Give 30 chest compressions (this may dislodge obstruction), then repeat TWO rescue breaths. Continue to give 30 compressions followed by two rescue breaths for one minute.

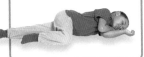

☎ **CALL AN AMBULANCE**

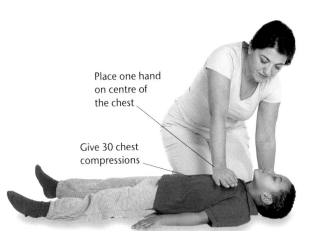

Place one hand on centre of the chest

Give 30 chest compressions

4 Continue alternating 30 chest compressions with two rescue breaths until help arrives, your child shows signs of recovery (*see box right*), or you are too exhausted to continue.

The recovery position

If your child shows signs of recovery such as coughing, opening his eyes, speaking or moving purposefully, and is breathing normally, place him in the recovery position (*see p.26*) and CALL AN AMBULANCE if not already done. Monitor breathing, pulse, and level of response until the ambulance arrives.

›› see also
- Checking vital signs, *p.14*
- Unresponsive child, *pp.22–27*

Breath holding

This is the result of rage and frustration. Your child is breath holding if he cries, then breathes in but does not breathe out. He may go blue in the face and stiff and may even become unresponsive momentarily.

see also

● Unresponsive child, pp.22–27

Blow into his face

1 Try to stay calm. Do not shake him or make a fuss. He will usually start breathing again spontaneously.

2 Try blowing directly into his face; this often results in a child starting to breathe again.

Hiccups

These are very common and usually only last for a few minutes, though often seem to go on for a long time. Children can become distressed.

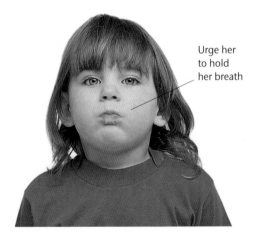

Urge her to hold her breath

1 Tell your child to sit still and to hold her breath for as long as she can. Then encourage her to breathe out slowly.

2 Get her to repeat this until hiccups have stopped.

Suffocation and strangulation

Strangulation results from a constriction around the child's neck that prevents breathing. Suffocation occurs when there is an obstruction over the mouth or nose, a weight on the child's chest or abdomen preventing normal breathing, or because the child is inhaling smoke- or fume-filled air, which prevents oxygen entering the lungs.

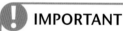

> ! **IMPORTANT**
> - **If** your child is hanging, support his body while you remove or cut the rope or cord.
> - **If** your child is not breathing, begin CPR immediately.

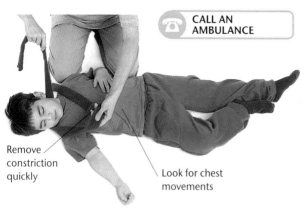

Remove constriction quickly

Look for chest movements

☎ **CALL AN AMBULANCE**

1 Remove the obstruction quickly. Use scissors to cut constriction if necessary. Breathing may restart.

2 Open your child's airway and check his breathing. If he is breathing, place him in the recovery position.

> » *see also*
> - Unresponsive baby, *pp.19–21*
> - Unresponsive child, *pp.22–27*

Fume inhalation

Fume, gas, and smoke inhalation requires urgent medical attention as the fumes prevent the child breathing in oxygen. Carbon monoxide prevents tissues taking up oxygen from air breathed in.

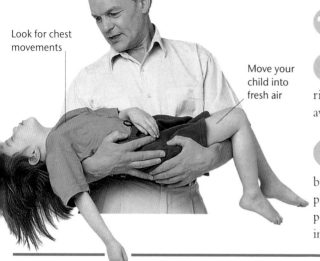

Look for chest movements

Move your child into fresh air

☎ **CALL AN AMBULANCE**

1 Ensure that you do not put yourself at risk. Then carry your child away from danger area.

2 Open her airway and check her breathing. If breathing, place her in the recovery position, and treat any injuries found.

> ! **IMPORTANT**
> - **Do not** enter the area if fumes, gas, carbon monoxide, or smoke are still present. CALL FIRE SERVICE and AMBULANCE.
> - **If** your child is not breathing, begin CPR immediately.

> » *see also*
> - Burns and scalds, *p.52*
> - Unresponsive baby, *pp.19–21*
> - Unresponsive child, *pp.22–27*

⚠ IMPORTANT

● **Do not put** your fingers in the child's throat – it could cause the throat muscles to go into spasm.

● **If** the attack is severe or prolonged, CALL AN AMBULANCE.

● **If** the attack is severe there is a risk that he is suffering from a rare croup-like condition called epiglottitis. Suspect this if your child has a high temperature and is obviously in distress. CALL AN AMBULANCE.

Croup

This condition is caused by a viral infection. It can be alarming and often occurs at night, but usually passes quickly. Your child will have difficulty breathing, and a short, distinctve barking cough when he breathes in. He may be making a crowing or whistling noise. In a severe attack, he may use muscles around his nose, neck, and upper arms in his attempts to breathe and he may have blue-tinged skin.

1 Help your child into a comfortable breathing position. Sit him up in bed, propped by pillows or sit him on your lap supporting his back. Reassure him.

2 Stay calm – if you panic it could frighten the child, which can worsen the attack.

SEEK MEDICAL ADVICE

3 Stay with the child and monitor his breathing, pulse, and level of response *(see p.14)* until he has recovered.

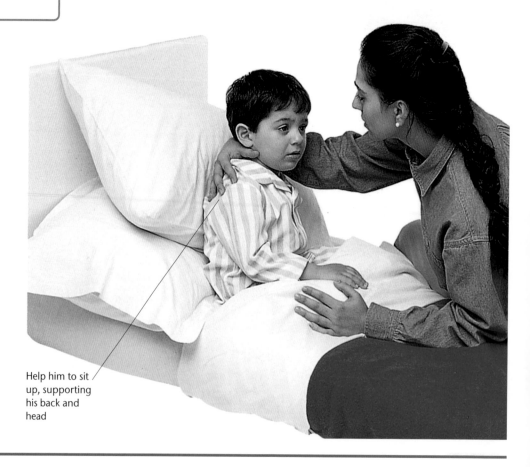

Help him to sit up, supporting his back and head

Asthma

If your child suffers from asthma, familiarise her with her medication so that she knows how to use it in an attack. You can recognise an attack if your child: has difficulty breathing and is coughing; is wheezing especially when breathing *out;* is distressed and anxious. She may also be tired by efforts to breathe and have a bluish tinge to face and lips.

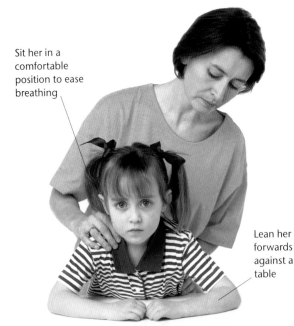

Sit her in a comfortable position to ease breathing

Lean her forwards against a table

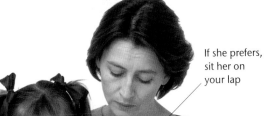

If she prefers, sit her on your lap

1 Give your child her usual dose of the reliever medication as soon as an attack starts, *see right.* Stay calm and reassure her. Tell her to breathe slowly and deeply.

2 Help your child to relax. Sit her down in a comfortable position for breathing. This could be leaning forwards with her arms resting on a table, or if she prefers sit her on your lap. Ensure the room is well-ventilated and smoke-free.

3 If the attack does not ease within a few minutes, give her 1-2 puffs from her medication every two minutes until she has had 10 puffs.

4 If the attack still does not ease,

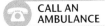 **CALL AN AMBULANCE**

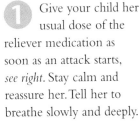

> **! IMPORTANT**
> ● **If** it is a first attack, CALL AN AMBULANCE.
>
> ● **If** the attack is severe, the medication has no effect, the child is exhausted, breathlessness makes talking difficult, and/or skin has a bluish tinge CALL AN AMBULANCE.

Using medication

Give your child her medication as soon as an attack starts. Make sure you give her the reliever inhaler – this has a blue cap. Usually if a child has an inhaler she will also have a spacer device to use with it, so use that as well as it's easier to take in the medication. Follow the directions carefully.

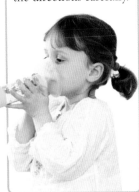

! IMPORTANT

- **Do not** move your child unnecessarily.

- **Do not** give your child anything to drink or eat as he may need an anaesthetic. If he is thirsty, just moisten his lips with water.

- **If** you suspect a broken leg only raise the uninjured leg.

Shock

The most likely cause is serious bleeding or a severe burn or scald – injuries that must be treated without delay. There could be internal bleeding if shock develops with no visible injury. Early signs are: pale, cold, and sweaty skin, tinged with grey; rapid pulse becoming weaker; shallow, fast breathing. As it develops he will: be restless, yawning, and sighing; be very thirsty; eventually he will be unresponsive.

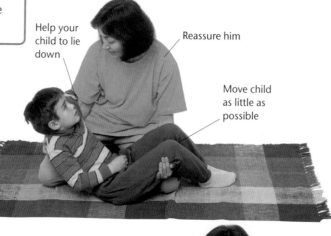

Help your child to lie down

Reassure him

Move child as little as possible

1 Treat any obvious injury. Help your child to lie down flat, on a blanket or rug if possible to protect him from the cold. Stay calm and reassure him.

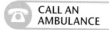

CALL AN AMBULANCE

2 Keep your child's head low; don't put a pillow under it. Carefully raise your child's legs above the level of his heart to help blood flow to the vital organs; support them on pillows, a chair, or a pile of books padded with a cushion.

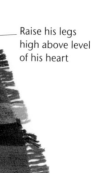

Head must be kept low

Raise his legs high above level of his heart

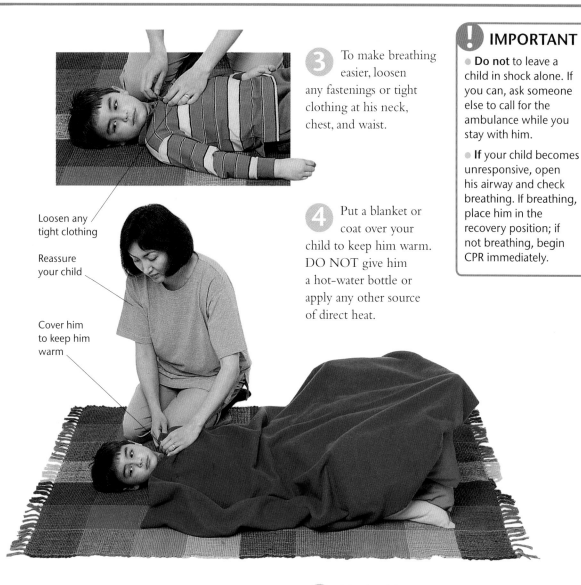

Loosen any
tight clothing

Reassure
your child

Cover him
to keep him
warm

③ To make breathing easier, loosen any fastenings or tight clothing at his neck, chest, and waist.

④ Put a blanket or coat over your child to keep him warm. DO NOT give him a hot-water bottle or apply any other source of direct heat.

! **IMPORTANT**

● **Do not** to leave a child in shock alone. If you can, ask someone else to call for the ambulance while you stay with him.

● **If** your child becomes unresponsive, open his airway and check breathing. If breathing, place him in the recovery position; if not breathing, begin CPR immediately.

Check his pulse rate, and note whether it is strong or weak, regular or irregular

⑤ Monitor his breathing, pulse, and level of response while you wait for the ambulance. Encourage him to talk or answer questions to help you assess any change in his condition. Make a note of any changes and tell the ambulance personnel.

》 *see also*
● Severe bleeding, *p.38*
● Burns and scalds, *p.52*
● Unresponsive baby, *pp.19–21*
● Unresponsive child, *pp.22–27*

Severe bleeding

Any incident that results in severe bleeding can be very distressing for you and your child. If it is not controlled quickly a life-threatening condition known as shock will develop. Large wounds may also need stitches.

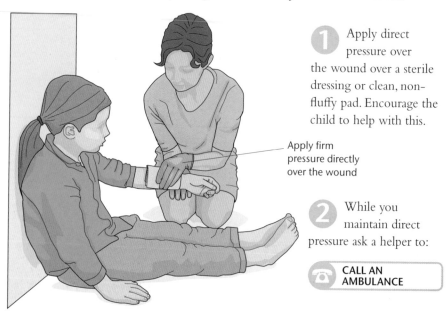

1 Apply direct pressure over the wound over a sterile dressing or clean, non-fluffy pad. Encourage the child to help with this.

Apply firm pressure directly over the wound

2 While you maintain direct pressure ask a helper to:

☎ CALL AN AMBULANCE

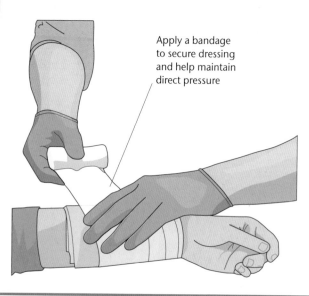

Apply a bandage to secure dressing and help maintain direct pressure

3 Secure the dressing with a bandage that is firm enough to maintain pressure, but not so tight that it affects the circulation beyond the bandage. Check the circulation in the hand or foot by pressing the nail. If colour does not return straightaway the bandage is too tight; remove it and reapply more loosely.

⟫ see also

● Check circulation, p.105

● Dressings, p.104

● Embedded object, p.40

● Shock, p.36

● Triangular bandages, p.106

4 Shock is likely to develop if bleeding is severe. Supporting your child's arm and maintaining pressure, help her to lie down on a blanket. Raise her legs above the level of her heart. Cover her with another blanket to keep her warm.

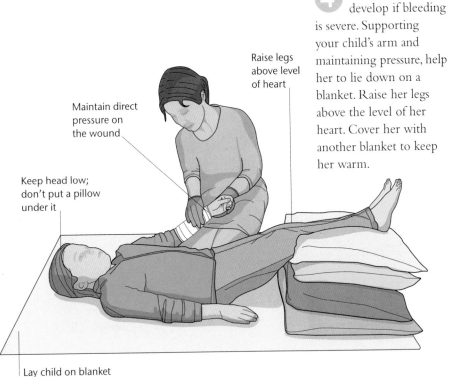

Maintain direct pressure on the wound

Raise legs above level of heart

Keep head low; don't put a pillow under it

Lay child on blanket to protect from cold

When bleeding stops

If the bleeding has stopped and there is no risk of shock, help the child to sit down and support an injured hand or arm in an elevation sling for extra comfort on the way to hospital.

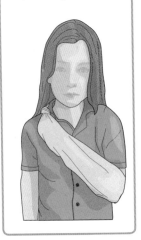

5 If bleeding shows through the first dressing put another pad on top of the first and secure with a bandage. If bleeding continues, direct pressure may not be over the right point. Remove both pads and start again making sure the new pad is over the wound. Check circulation regularly; loosen and reapply bandage if necessary.

Put a second pad directly over first one and secure with a bandage

6 Monitor child's breathing, pulse, and level of response while waiting for emergency help to arrive.

! IMPORTANT

- **Do not** try to remove, or dislodge, objects that are embedded in a wound as you may cause further damage and bleeding.

Bandaging around larger objects

If the object is very big, build up padding either side, then bandage above and below the object instead of over the top.

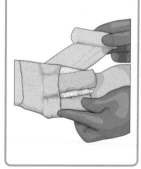

» see also

- Severe bleeding, *p.38*

Embedded object

If an object such as a piece of glass becomes stuck in a wound, it is serious as it may be plugging the wound, preventing bleeding. Do not remove it. Protect it with padding and bandages and get medical help.

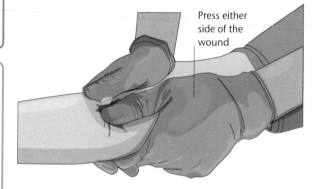

Press either side of the wound

1 Help your child to lie down and keep him calm. If necessary apply pressure on either side of the object – pushing the edges of the wound together – to help control bleeding.

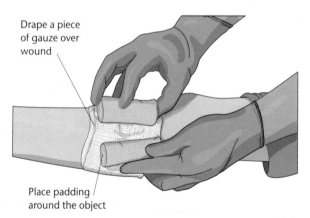

Drape a piece of gauze over wound

Place padding around the object

2 Loosely drape some gauze over the wound and object to minimise the risk of infection. If the object is small, build up padding so that it is slightly higher than the embedded object; spare roller bandages are ideal for this. If the object is large, *see box left*.

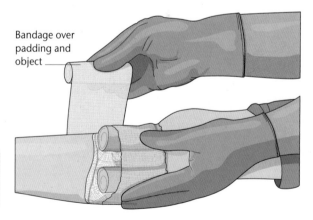

Bandage over padding and object

3 Secure padding in place by bandaging over it, being careful not to press down on the embedded object.

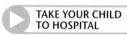
TAKE YOUR CHILD TO HOSPITAL

OR

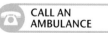
CALL AN AMBULANCE

Cuts and grazes

Children can be very upset by the tiniest graze. Reassure your child and wash the wound. Covering the wound with a plaster keeps it clean and often makes the child feel better.

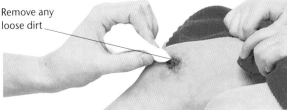

Sit child down

Wash graze

1 Help your child to sit down and reassure her. Gently wash the graze with soap and water using a gauze pad or a very soft brush. If the wound is very dirty rinse under cold running water.

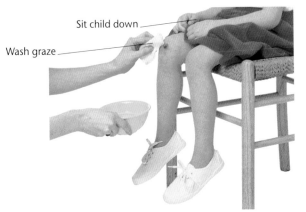

Remove any loose dirt

2 Try to remove any loose particles of dirt or gravel with the corner of a piece of gauze or cold running water. This may cause slight bleeding.

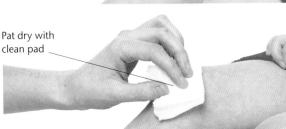

Pat dry with clean pad

3 Apply direct pressure with a clean pad to stop any bleeding. Pat the wound dry with clean pieces of gauze.

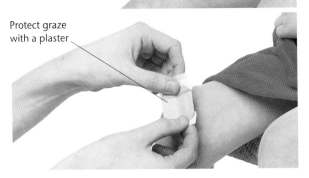

Protect graze with a plaster

4 Cover the cut or graze with a plaster that has a pad large enough to cover the wound and the area around it.

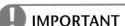

! IMPORTANT

- **Do not** clean or cover cuts with cotton wool or any fluffy material; it may stick to the wound and will delay healing.

- **Loosen** particles of dirt by rinsing the wound under cold running water.

- **If** particles are embedded *see opposite* and TAKE YOUR CHILD TO HOSPITAL.

- **Check** that your child's tetanus immunisation is up to date.

Tetanus

This is a dangerous infection that is present in the soil. If it is transferred into a wound, tetanus germs release toxins (poisons) into the nervous system. Tetanus is best prevented through vaccination. Babies receive this as part of their immunisation programme. Every child should be given a tetanus booster before starting school.

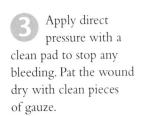

see also

- Infected wound, *p.42*

Tetanus

This is a dangerous infection caused by a bacterium present in the soil. If these bacteria are transferred into a wound, they may multiply and release toxins (poisons) into the nervous system. Tetanus is best prevented through vaccination. Babies receive this as part of their immunisation programme. Every child should be given a tetanus booster before starting school.

Infected wound

A wound is infected if there is: increasing pain and soreness; swelling, redness, and a feeling of heat around the injury; pus within, or oozing from, the wound. If infection is advanced there may also be swelling and tenderness in the glands in the neck, armpit, or groin, and possible faint red trails on the skin leading to these glands. In addition there may be signs of fever (sweating, thirst, shivering, and lethargy).

1 Cover the wound with an adhesive dressing or clean non-fluffy pad or sterile dressing secured in place with a bandage.

2 Raise and support the infected wound. Reassure the child.

☎ SEEK MEDICAL ADVICE

3 If there are signs and symptoms advanced infection,

▷ TAKE YOUR CHILD TO HOSPITAL

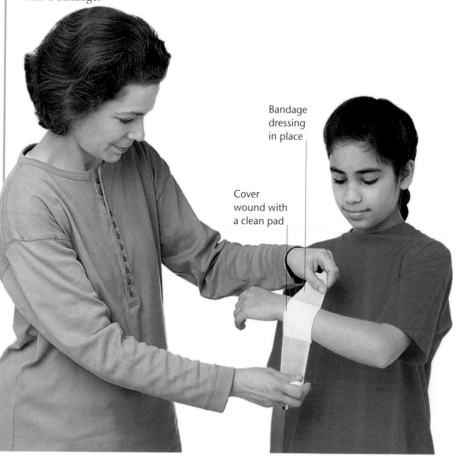

Bandage dressing in place

Cover wound with a clean pad

Blisters

If a blister is caused by friction (for example, a badly fitting shoe) treat as here. You can buy special padded blister plasters.

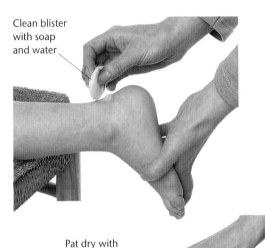

Clean blister with soap and water

1 Clean the blister thoroughly with soap and water. Rinse it with clean water.

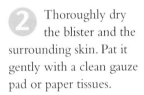

Pat dry with clean pad

2 Thoroughly dry the blister and the surrounding skin. Pat it gently with a clean gauze pad or paper tissues.

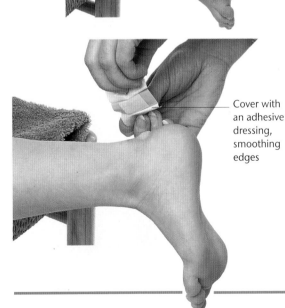

Cover with an adhesive dressing, smoothing edges

3 Ideally cover it with a blister plaster if you have one, if not a normal one will do. The plaster needs to have a pad large enough to cover the entire blister. Make sure the edges are smooth, to prevent another blister developing.

 see also

● Burns and scalds, *p.52*

Eye wound

This type of wound is serious because of the risk of damage to the child's sight. Injury can scar the surface of the eye or lead to infection.

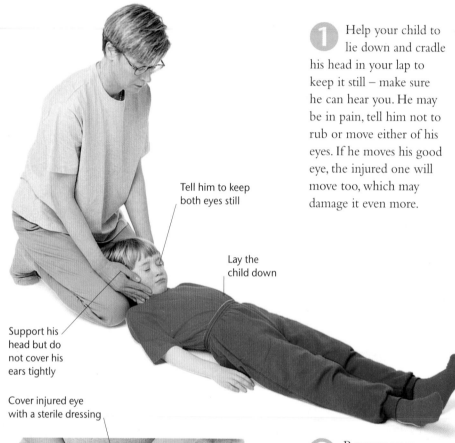

Tell him to keep both eyes still

Lay the child down

Support his head but do not cover his ears tightly

1 Help your child to lie down and cradle his head in your lap to keep it still – make sure he can hear you. He may be in pain, tell him not to rub or move either of his eyes. If he moves his good eye, the injured one will move too, which may damage it even more.

Cover injured eye with a sterile dressing

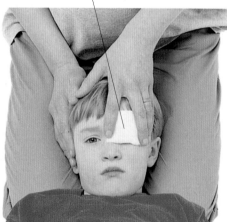

2 Reassure your child and then cover the injured eye with a sterile dressing. Hold the dressing in place until you get medical help.

3 Keep him lying on his back.

⟫ see also

● Chemical burn to eye, p.56

● Object in eye, p.76

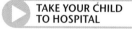

▶ TAKE YOUR CHILD TO HOSPITAL

Nosebleed

Children get nosebleeds from a blow to the nose, or from picking it. Bleeding usually stops quickly, but it can alarm young children.

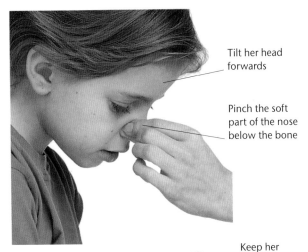

Tilt her head forwards

Pinch the soft part of the nose below the bone

1 Help your child to sit down with her head well forwards. Ask her to breathe through her mouth, then pinch the fleshy part of her nose for 10 minutes. Then release the pressure.

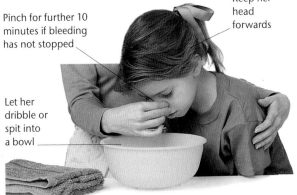

Keep her head forwards

Pinch for further 10 minutes if bleeding has not stopped

Let her dribble or spit into a bowl

2 Tell your child to spit out any excess fluid in her mouth. If the bleeding has not stopped, pinch it again for another 10 minutes, then release pressure. If the nose is still bleeding, pinch it again for up to 10 minutes.

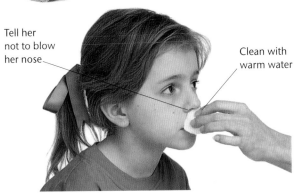

Tell her not to blow her nose

Clean with warm water

3 Once the bleeding has stopped, use some cotton wool dipped in lukewarm water to clean your child's face. Advise her to rest and not to blow her nose. If your child picks at (or blows) her nose within the next few hours, the bleeding may start again.

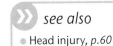

» see also
● Head injury, *p.60*

Ear wound

Outer ear wounds can bleed profusely, which can be alarming. If blood is coming from inside the ear, check that your child has not inserted something into it. If bleeding follows a head injury, CALL AN AMBULANCE.

! IMPORTANT

● **If** the bleeding follows a head injury and there is blood or watery blood-stained fluid draining from the ear, CALL AN AMBULANCE.

● **If** the injury is caused by an earring being ripped out, your child may need stitches. TAKE YOUR CHILD TO HOSPITAL.

Bleeding from inside the ear

Help your child into a semi-upright position, with his head tilted towards the injured side to allow blood to drain away. Put an absorbent pad over the ear and bandage it lightly in place. Do not plug the ear. SEEK MEDICAL ADVICE.

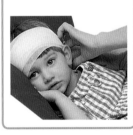

» *see also*

● Head injury, *p.60*
● Object in ear, *p.77*

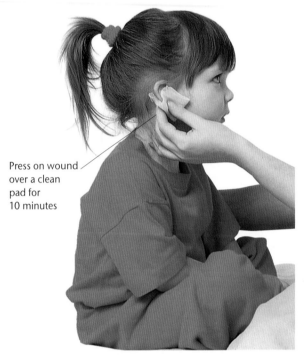

Press on wound over a clean pad for 10 minutes

1 Help your child to sit down and gently pinch the wound with your thumb and forefinger over a clean piece of gauze. Keep pressing for 10 minutes.

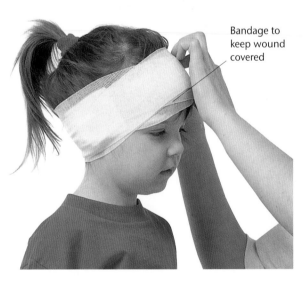

Bandage to keep wound covered

2 Cover the injured ear with a sterile dressing and lightly bandage it in place.

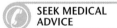

SEEK MEDICAL ADVICE

Mouth wound

These wounds can be the result of a child biting the inside of his mouth in a fall, for example, or from the loss of a tooth. Make sure your child does not inhale blood, as this can result in breathing problems.

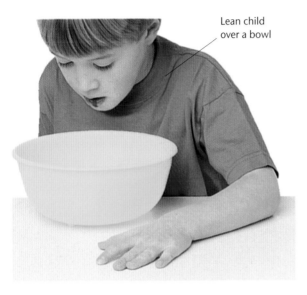

Lean child over a bowl

1 Help your child to sit down with his head over a bowl. Encourage him to spit out any blood.

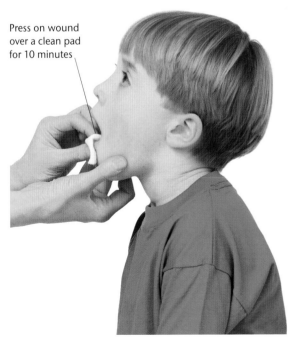

Press on wound over a clean pad for 10 minutes

2 Place a pad over the wound and pinch it between your thumb and forefinger, maintaining the pressure for 10 minutes. Your child may be able to do this for himself.

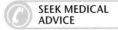

SEEK MEDICAL ADVICE

! IMPORTANT

● **Do not** wash out his mouth as this may disturb a blood clot.

● **If** he loses a tooth, it may be possible for a dentist to replant an "adult" tooth. Do not clean the tooth. Keep it moist by putting the tooth in milk or saliva TAKE YOUR CHILD TO THE DENTIST.

● **Ensure** a milk tooth has not been inhaled or swallowed. A dentist should check the gum.

Bleeding from tooth socket

Ask your child to sit down and support her jaw. Place a pad over the tooth socket, making sure that it is higher than the adjacent teeth. Tell her to bite hard on the pad. A younger child may need you to hold the pad in place.

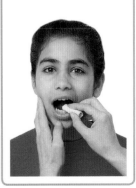

! IMPORTANT
● **Do not** use a tourniquet.

● **Get** to a hospital quickly. It may be possible to reattach an amputated part using microsurgery when both the child and the severed part reach the hospital in time.

● **Never** wash the severed part or allow it to come into direct contact with ice.

● **Do not** apply cotton wool to open wounds.

Care of the amputated part

Preserve the severed part until you get to hospital. Wrap it in kitchen film or a plastic bag, then in a soft fabric, such as a cotton handkerchief or piece of gauze. Place the wrapped part in a plastic bag filled with ice cubes; the part must not touch the ice. Put the whole package in another bag or container. Mark with the time of injury and the child's name then give it to the ambulance personnel.

Amputation

Whether a injury causes partial or total amputation, the limb can often be reattached. Your child will need an anaesthetic so don't give him anything to eat or drink because it will delay surgery.

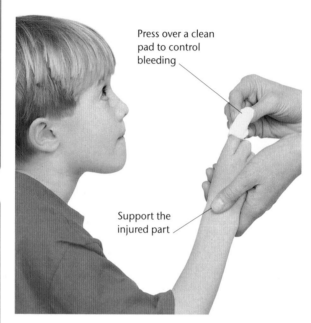

Press over a clean pad to control bleeding

Support the injured part

1 Control the blood loss by pressing firmly on the injury using a sterile dressing or clean pad. If necessary, treat for shock; help your child to lie down and raise his legs above his heart.

2 Bandage or tape the dressing firmly in place. You can cover a finger with a gauze finger bandage to protect it.

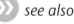

☎ CALL AN AMBULANCE

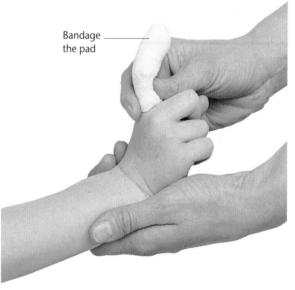

Bandage the pad

3 Tell the emergency services control it is an amputation. Monitor your child for signs of shock while waiting. If possible, put the severed part in a plastic bag and keep it cool, *see left*.

≫ *see also*
● Severe bleeding, *p.38*
● Shock, *p.36*

Internal bleeding

Suspect this when signs of shock develop without obvious blood loss. There may also be "pattern bruising" around the injury with marks from clothes or crushing objects. There could also be bleeding from orifices such as the nose or ear. Note what this looks like and keep a sample.

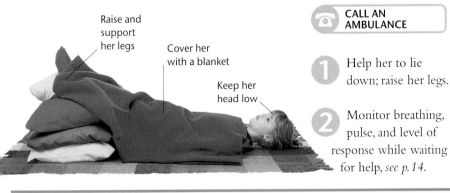

Raise and support her legs

Cover her with a blanket

Keep her head low

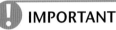
☎ **CALL AN AMBULANCE**

1 Help her to lie down; raise her legs.

2 Monitor breathing, pulse, and level of response while waiting for help, *see p.14.*

❗ IMPORTANT

● **If** the child is unresponsive, open her airway and check breathing. If breathing, place in the recovery position; if she is not breathing, begin CPR immediately.

» see also

● Shock, *p.36*
● Unresponsive baby, *pp.19–21*
● Unresponsive child, *pp.22–27*

Crush injury

A crush injury can be serious as it may cause internal bleeding and broken bones as well as open wounds.

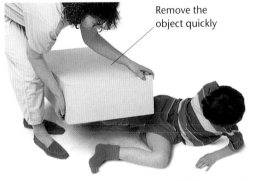

Remove the object quickly

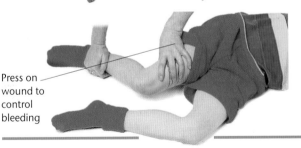

Press on wound to control bleeding

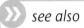
☎ **CALL AN AMBULANCE**

1 If the incident has only just happened, remove the heavy object from the child quickly.

2 Control any bleeding by pressing firmly on the wound, with your hand or a clean pad. Support the injured part, but do not move it.

❗ IMPORTANT

● **If** your child has been crushed for over 15 minutes, do not remove the object as it may cause toxic fluids from the damaged muscles to be released into the body. This increases the risk of shock.

● **If** you suspect broken bones, support the injury, but do not move your child unless he is in immediate danger and it is safe to do so. Watch for signs of shock while waiting for help.

» see also

● Severe bleeding, *p.38*
● Shock, *p.36*
● Leg injury, *p.64*

! IMPORTANT

● **Monitor** your child for signs of shock.

● **If** child becomes unresponsive, open his airway and check breathing. If breathing, place in the recovery position; if not breathing, begin CPR immediately.

● **If** you need to place him in the recovery position place him so that he is lying on his injured side to support his chest and help the good lung function.

Chest wound

A chest wound may cause severe internal injuries. The lungs are particularly vulnerable, and breathing problems, shock, and collapsed lungs may follow an injury. If the wound is not obviously bleeding, leave it exposed – don't cover it with a dresssing.

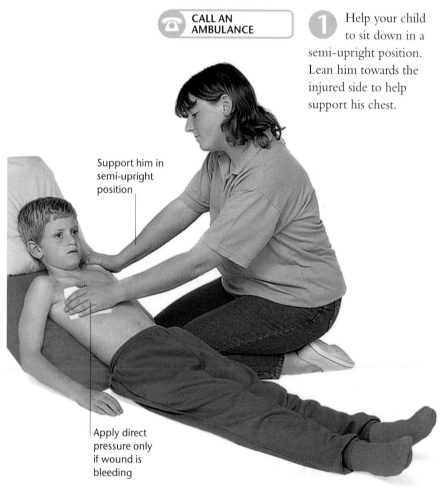

☎ **CALL AN AMBULANCE**

① Help your child to sit down in a semi-upright position. Lean him towards the injured side to help support his chest.

Support him in semi-upright position

Apply direct pressure only if wound is bleeding

》 see also

● Checking vital signs, *p.14*

● Severe bleeding, *p.38*

● Shock, *p.36*

● Unresponsive child, *pp.22–27*

② If the wound is obviously bleeding apply direct pressure with your hand – over a dressing if there's one available. Support the child in the same position until help arrives.

③ Monitor his breathing, pulse, and level of response while you wait for help to arrive.

Abdominal wound

A child with an abdominal wound is likely to develop the signs of shock. There is high risk of internal as well as external bleeding as internal organs may be damaged, so this is an emergency.

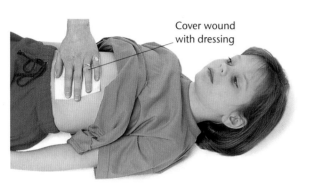

Cover wound with dressing

1 Help your child to lie down and loosen any tight clothing around her waist. Cover the injury with a large sterile dressing and apply pressure over the pad; the child may be able to help.

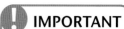

> **! IMPORTANT**
>
> ● **Monitor** your child for signs of shock.
>
> ● **If** your child becomes unresponsive, open her airway and check breathing. If breathing, place her in the recovery position, supporting her abdomen while you turn her. If she is not breathing, begin CPR immediately.

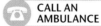
CALL AN AMBULANCE

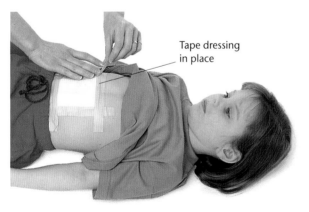

Tape dressing in place

2 Reassure your child. Raise and support her knees by placing a cushion under them – this eases the strain on the abdomen.

3 Secure the dressing lightly in place with tape; use hypoallergenic tape if possible.

4 Monitor her breathing, pulse, and level of response while you wait for help to arrive. Treat for shock if necessary. Continue to reassure her and watch for any change in her condition while waiting for help.

> **》 see also**
>
> ● Checking vital signs, *p.14*
>
> ● Severe bleeding, *p.38*
>
> ● Shock, *p.36*
>
> ● Unresponsive child, *pp.22–27*

Burns and scalds

Burns to the mouth and throat

Burns in this area are very serious as they cause swelling and inflammation of the air passages, giving a serious risk of suffocation. Act quickly. If necessary, loosen clothing from around her neck. If your child develops breathing difficulties, open her airway and check breathing. If she is not breathing begin CPR immediately. CALL AN AMBULANCE.

It is very important to cool the burn as quickly as possible to stop the burning and so minimise damage and reduce pain. You must always seek medical advice or take a child to hospital following any burn – however small – as there is a high risk of infection.

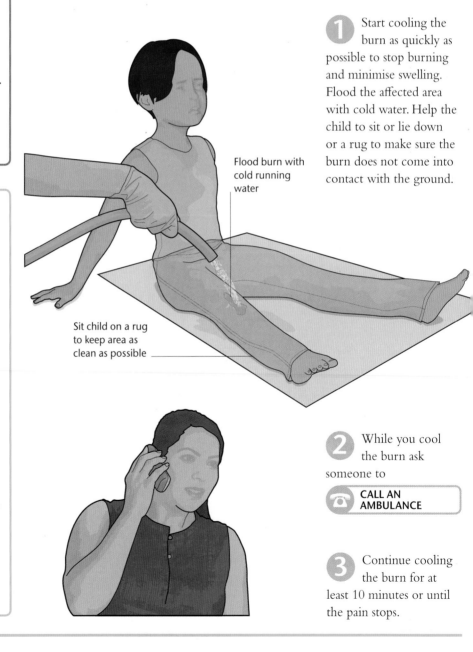

Flood burn with cold running water

Sit child on a rug to keep area as clean as possible

1 Start cooling the burn as quickly as possible to stop burning and minimise swelling. Flood the affected area with cold water. Help the child to sit or lie down or a rug to make sure the burn does not come into contact with the ground.

2 While you cool the burn ask someone to

☎ **CALL AN AMBULANCE**

3 Continue cooling the burn for at least 10 minutes or until the pain stops.

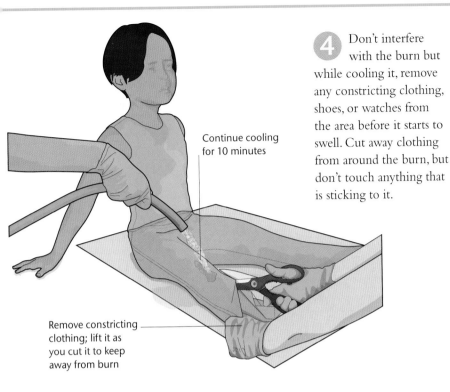

Continue cooling for 10 minutes

Remove constricting clothing; lift it as you cut it to keep away from burn

4 Don't interfere with the burn but while cooling it, remove any constricting clothing, shoes, or watches from the area before it starts to swell. Cut away clothing from around the burn, but don't touch anything that is sticking to it.

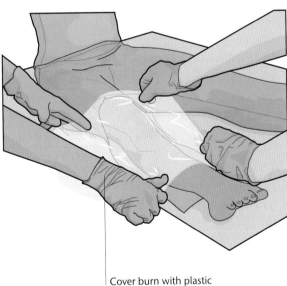

Cover burn with plastic kitchen film to protect from infection

5 Once the burn is cooled cover it with plastic kitchen film. Lay it lengthways along the limb; don't wrap film around a limb as it will swell. Monitor breathing, pulse, and level of response while you are waiting for help to arrive.

》 *see also*
● Checking vital signs, *p.14*
● Fire, *p.11*
● Shock, *p.36*
● Unresponsive baby, *pp.19–21*
● Unresponsive child, *pp.22–27*

❗ IMPORTANT

● **Do not** remove any clothing or material that is sticking to the burnt area as this may cause further injury.

● **If** you have no kitchen film use a sterile dressing or any clean non-fluffy material.

● **Do not** give your child anything to eat or drink as an anaesthetic may be needed.

● **If** the child becomes unresponsive, open airway and check breathing. If breathing, place in the recovery position; if not breathing, begin CPR immediately. CALL AN AMBULANCE.

Using a plastic bag

You can use a clean plastic bag to protect an injured hand or foot. Secure it loosely with a piece of tape that is applied to the bag; don't put tape on the child's skin.

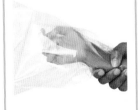

Electrical burn

An electric shock from a low-voltage source can result in burns. These may occur at both the point of entry and the point of exit of the current.

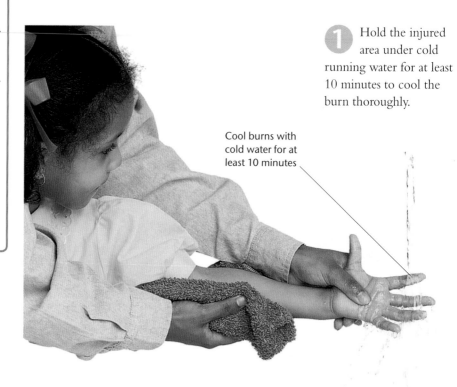

1 Hold the injured area under cold running water for at least 10 minutes to cool the burn thoroughly.

Cool burns with cold water for at least 10 minutes

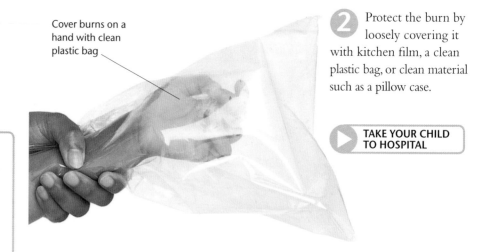

Cover burns on a hand with clean plastic bag

2 Protect the burn by loosely covering it with kitchen film, a clean plastic bag, or clean material such as a pillow case.

▶ **TAKE YOUR CHILD TO HOSPITAL**

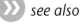 *see also*

● Electrical injury, *p.12*

● Unresponsive baby, *pp.19–21*

● Unresponsive child, *p.22–27*

Chemical burn to skin

Chemical burns can be caused by household agents such as oven cleaner or paint stripper. These burns are serious and there will be: fierce, stinging pain, redness or staining, followed by blistering and peeling of skin.

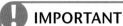

IMPORTANT

- **Seek** medical advice for all burns to children.

- **Note** the name of the substance that caused the burn and give the information to the hospital staff.

- **Always** wear protective gloves when treating your child, and beware of chemical fumes.

- **Don't** wrap kitchen film right around a limb as the injury is likely to swell.

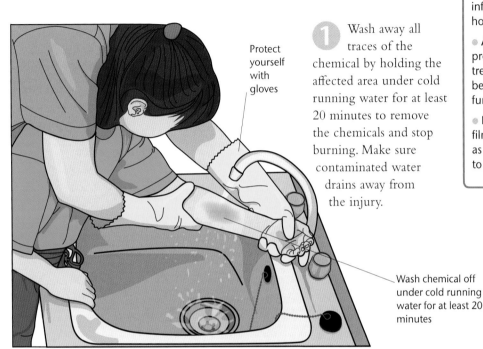

Protect yourself with gloves

1 Wash away all traces of the chemical by holding the affected area under cold running water for at least 20 minutes to remove the chemicals and stop burning. Make sure contaminated water drains away from the injury.

Wash chemical off under cold running water for at least 20 minutes

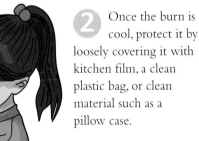

Cover burn loosely

2 Once the burn is cool, protect it by loosely covering it with kitchen film, a clean plastic bag, or clean material such as a pillow case.

▷ **TAKE YOUR CHILD TO HOSPITAL**

OR

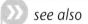 **CALL AN AMBULANCE**

›› see also

- Chemical burn to eye, *p.56*
- Fume inhalation, *p.33*
- Swallowed chemicals, *p.57*

! IMPORTANT

• **Do not** let your child touch his eye. The eye will be shut in spasm and pain, so gently pull the eyelids open.

Chemical burn to eye

Splashes of chemicals in the eye can cause scarring or even blindness. Your child may have a chemical burn if he complains of fierce pain in the eye; he has difficulty opening the affected eye; the surface of the eye is watery; there is redness and swelling in and around the eye.

Using a jug of water

If you can't hold your child under a tap, you may find it easier to use a jug to pour water over the affected eye. Get a helper to support the child with her head tilted down and to one side. Avoid splashing the "good" eye with the contaminated water.

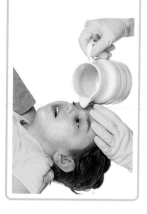

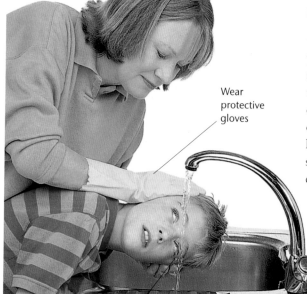

Wear protective gloves

Rinse eye with cold water for 10 minutes

1 Protect yourself from the chemical with rubber gloves. Hold your child's head over a sink, with the "good" eye uppermost. Gently run cold water over the contaminated eye for at least 10 minutes. Make sure that both sides of the eyelid are thoroughly washed and that the contaminated water drains away from your child's face.

Cover eye with clean pad

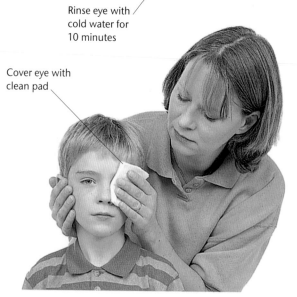

2 Once the injured eye is thoroughly washed, cover it with a large sterile dressing. Hold the dressing in place until you get medical aid.

▶ **TAKE YOUR CHILD TO HOSPITAL**

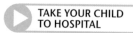

OR

☎ **CALL AN AMBULANCE**

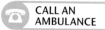

Swallowed chemicals

If you think your child has swallowed a poison, try to find out what, when, and how much she has taken. Be aware too that some chemicals also give off dangerous fumes.

! IMPORTANT

● **Do not** try to make your child vomit as this can cause further harm.

● **If** your child becomes unresponsive, open her airway and check breathing. If breathing, place her in the recovery position; if not breathing, begin CPR immediately.

● **If** you need to give rescue breaths and there are chemicals on the child's mouth, protect yourself by using a face shield or pocket mask.

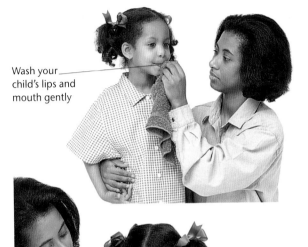

Wash your child's lips and mouth gently

1 Wipe away any residual chemical from around your child's mouth and face.

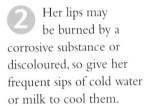

Help her take sips of cold water

2 Her lips may be burned by a corrosive substance or discoloured, so give her frequent sips of cold water or milk to cool them.

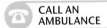

☎ CALL AN AMBULANCE

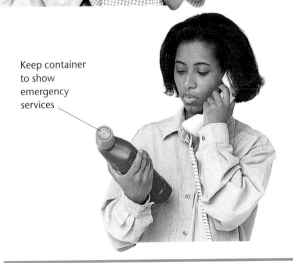

Keep container to show emergency services

3 Find out what chemical your child swallowed and when, and if possible how much, then tell the emergency services when you make the call. This will help them determine the correct treatment.

≫ see also

● Chemical burn to eye, *opposite*

● Fume inhalation, *p.33*

● Unresponsive baby, *pp.19–21*

● Unresponsive child, *pp.22–27*

! IMPORTANT

- **Do not** make your child sick as it can cause more harm. If he is sick, give a sample to the ambulance personnel.

- **Even** a small amount of alcohol may harm a young child.

- **If** your child is drowsy or becomes unresponsive, open airway and check breathing. If breathing, place him in the recovery position; if not breathing, begin CPR immediately.

⟫ see also

- Unresponsive baby, pp.19–21

- Unresponsive child, pp.22–27

Drug or alcohol poisoning

If your child has taken medication the container may be nearby. If he drank alcohol there may be a smell of alcohol and he may be staggering and be sick. He may also have: a flushed and moist face; slurred speech; deep noisy breathing; a bounding pulse.

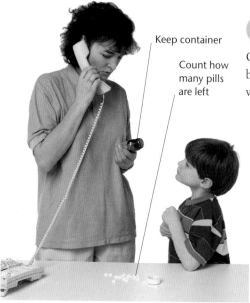

Keep container

Count how many pills are left

1 Try to find out what he has taken, when, and how much. Check the label on the medicine bottle and tell the emergency services when you ring.

☏ CALL AN AMBULANCE

2 If he drank alcohol, let your child rest where you can watch him while waiting for the ambulance. Give him a bowl in case he is sick. If he falls asleep, try to wake him to make sure he can be easily roused.

! IMPORTANT

- **Do not** make your child vomit. This can cause further harm. If he does vomit, keep a sample.

Plant poisoning

Many plants are poisonous in large quantities. Small pieces or one or two berries are unlikely to be fatal but can cause stomach upset.

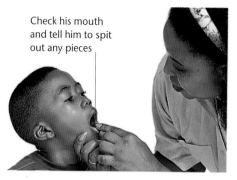

Check his mouth and tell him to spit out any pieces

1 Try to find out what your child ate, when, and how much – keep a sample.

☏ SEEK MEDICAL ADVICE

2 Look inside your child's mouth. Pick out any remaining pieces of plant or berries.

Scalp wound

This type of wound can bleed profusely. If the wound was caused by a blow to the child's head, watch for any change in her condition, especially her level of response, while waiting for the ambulance.

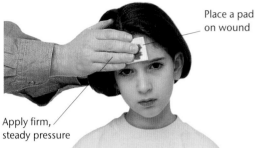

Place a pad on wound

Apply firm, steady pressure

1 Cover the injury with a clean pad or sterile dressing that is larger than the wound. Press firmly on the pad and the wound to control the bleeding. Place another pad on top, if necessary, and keep pressing on the wound.

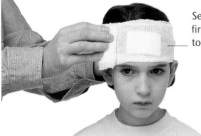

Secure bandage firmly but not too tightly

2 Bandage the dressing firmly in place. If the bleeding continues, apply pressure again with your hand.

3 Help your child to lie down with her head and shoulders slightly raised.

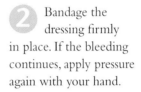

📞 CALL AN AMBULANCE

4 Check breathing, pulse, and level of response while waiting for help *(see p.14)*.

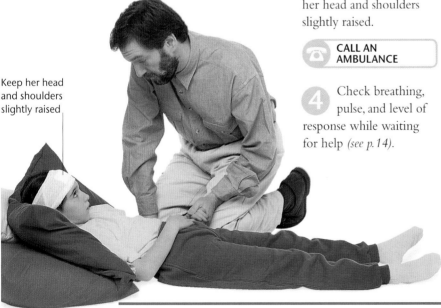

Keep her head and shoulders slightly raised

❗ IMPORTANT

● **If** blood continues to seep through the two dressings, remove both pads and apply a new dressing.

● **If** your child becomes unresponsive, open her airway and check breathing. If breathing, place in the recovery position; if not breathing, begin CPR immediately.

» see also

● Head injury, *p.60*

● Severe bleeding, *p.38*

● Shock, *p.36*

● Unresponsive baby, *pp.19–21*

● Unresponsive child, *pp.22–27*

! IMPORTANT

● **Never** shake a baby or child to assess her reactions.

● **If** a head injury occurs during a sporting activity, do not allow your child to play on until she has been asessed by a healthcare professional.

Signs of worsening head injury

Seek urgent medical advice if after a head injury you notice any of the following in your child.

● She becomes disoriented and/or increasingly drowsy;

● She complains of double vision;

● She is vomiting;

● She complains of a persistent headache;

● She is confused, with loss of memory, dizziness;

● She has difficulty speaking and/or walking and problems with balance;

● She suffers a seizure.

Head injury

If your child has a minor bump to the head, she may simply have a bruise with no other sign of injury. If, however, the child has suffered a more serious blow, the brain can be shaken inside the skull and she may be dazed or temporarily unresponsive, but will suffer no lasting damage to the brain – this is concussion. Your child may have a headache, feel dizzy, complain of nausea, and may not remember what happened.

If there has been severe blow to the head there may be bleeding or swelling within the skull that can press on the brain – known as compression, this is a serious condition. A child may seem unaffected at first, but as time goes by (minutes, hours, or even days) her condition can worsen and so it is very important to watch her and monitor her condition looking for signs of a worsening head injury (*see box left*).

1 If the child is dazed, help her to lie down on the floor (protect her from the cold). Don't sit her on a chair as she may fall off and hurt herself.

2 If your child was "knocked out" even briefly,

SEEK MEDICAL ADVICE

3 Make her rest and watch her closely. Check her for signs of a worsening head injury, *left*, reassure her and stay with her. If she does not recover completely or shows any sign of deterioration,

CALL AN AMBULANCE

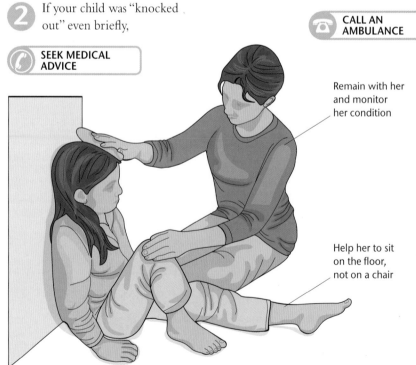

Remain with her and monitor her condition

Help her to sit on the floor, not on a chair

Checking a child's level of response

Your child could be awake following an injury, completely unresponsive, or somewhere between the two. She may deteriorate over minutes, hours, or even days. It is important to assess her condition and monitor any changes so that you can tell the ambulance personnel or hospital staff.

● Is she alert? Are her eyes open and does she respond normally when you talk to her?

● Does she only respond to voice by answering simple questions or obeying instructions? Does she open her eyes?

● Does she respond only to pain? For example by opening her eyes if you flick her foot or tap her shoulder.

● Is she completely unresponsive?

Note down any response or change of response, and the time.

IMPORTANT

● **Suspect** skull fracture if the level of response is impaired, there is blood or blood-stained watery fluid coming from the nose or ear; there is a soft area on the scalp; blood showing on the white of the eye; and/or distortion of the face or head.

● **Remember** there's a possibility of a spinal injury with any head injury.

If your child becomes unresponsive

Do not move your child as there could be an associated back or neck injury and moving her could result in damage to the brain or spinal cord.

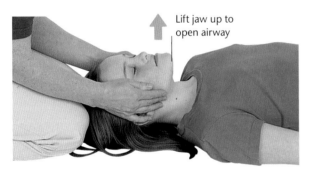

Lift jaw up to open airway

1 Kneel behind her head and rest your elbows on the ground or your knees. Open her airway using the jaw thrust: place one hand on either side of her face, with your fingertips on the angles of her jaw. Gently lift the jaw up to open the airway (don't tilt her head back).

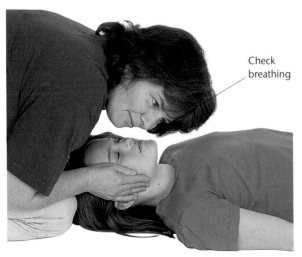

Check breathing

2 Check her breathing. If she is breathing continue to support her jaw to keep the airway open. If she is not breathing, begin CPR immediately. Ask someone else to

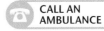
CALL AN AMBULANCE

see also

● Checking vital signs, *p.14*
● Cold packs, *p.108*
● Scalp wound, *p.59*
● Spine injury, *p.63*
● Unresponsive baby, *pp.19–21*
● Unresponsive child, *pp.22–27*

! IMPORTANT

● **If** pinching her nose hurts too much, simply ask her to sit forward over the bowl and give her a soft pad or towel to soak up the blood.

● **If** your child becomes unresponsive, open airway and check her breathing. If breathing, place in the recovery position; if not breathing, begin CPR immediately. CALL AN AMBULANCE.

» see also

● Nosebleed, p.45

● Unresponsive baby, pp.19–21

● Unresponsive child, pp.22–27

Nose/cheekbone injury

The main risk with fractures to the nose or cheek bones is that the swelling can affect the air passages causing breathing problems. There may also be bleeding from the child's nose or mouth.

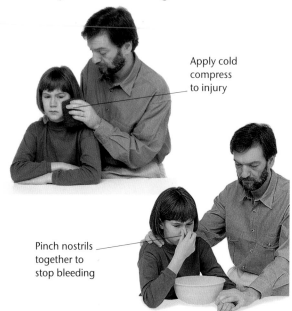

Apply cold compress to injury

Pinch nostrils together to stop bleeding

1 Help your child to sit down and apply a cold pack (*see p. 108*) to the injured area to help minimise the swelling. Hold the cold pack in place for about 20 minutes.

2 If your child's nose is bleeding, ask her to sit with her head well forward and to pinch the fleshy part of her nose to help control bleeding.

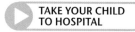

▶ **TAKE YOUR CHILD TO HOSPITAL**

! IMPORTANT

● **If** your child becomes unresponsive, open airway and check her breathing. If breathing, place in the recovery position; if not breathing, begin CPR. CALL AN AMBULANCE.

» see also

● Unresponsive baby, pp.19–21

● Unresponsive child, p.22–27

Jaw injury

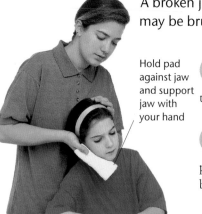

Hold pad against jaw and support jaw with your hand

A broken jaw it will be tender and swollen, and may be bruised. Her teeth may be out of line.

1 Help your child to sit with head well forwards. Tell her to spit out any loose teeth and not to swallow any blood or saliva.

2 Hold a soft pad firmly under her injured jaw, and support it in this position until you get to hospital. Do not bandage the pad in place in case she vomits.

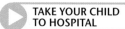

▶ **TAKE YOUR CHILD TO HOSPITAL**

Spine injury

If a child lands on his neck or back in a fall or falls awkwardly and complains of back pain or tingling in any part of his body, suspect spine injury. Support him in the position found to prevent further damage.

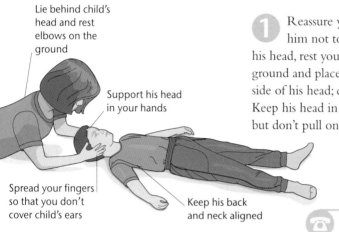

Lie behind child's head and rest elbows on the ground

Support his head in your hands

Spread your fingers so that you don't cover child's ears

Keep his back and neck aligned

1 Reassure your child and tell him not to move. Lie behind his head, rest your elbows on the ground and place your hands either side of his head; don't cover his ears. Keep his head in line with his spine, but don't pull on his neck.

☎ **CALL AN AMBULANCE**

Maintain head support

2 Keep his head and neck supported in the same position until help arrives. Ask someone to put rolled blankets or towels around his neck and shoulders for extra support.

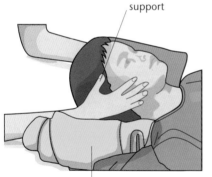

Place rolled blankets around his head and shoulders

Rolled blankets and towels provide extra support

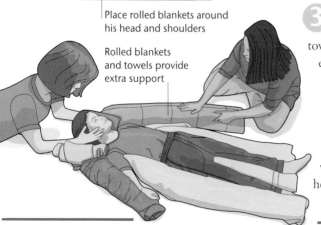

3 Ask your helper to arrange rolled towels or blankets along either side of his body while you continue to keep his head steady. Monitor breathing, pulse, and level of response while waiting for help to arrive.

! IMPORTANT

● **Do not** move the injured child from the position in which you find him unless his life is in danger.

● **If** you do have to move him, take care not to twist or bend the neck or spine.

● **If** your child becomes unresponsive, open airway using the jaw thrust technique (*see p.61*) and check breathing. If breathing, maintain the jaw thrust and keep the head, neck, and spine aligned; if not breathing, begin CPR immediately. CALL AN AMBULANCE.

» see also

● Checking vital signs, *p.14*

● Head injury, *p.60*

● Unresponsive baby, *pp.19–21*

● Unresponsive child, *pp.22–27*

» *see also*
● Shock, *p.36*

Pelvic injury

If your child has a broken pelvis she will be unable to stand, with pain around the hip and groin, and possible bleeding from the urinary orifice.

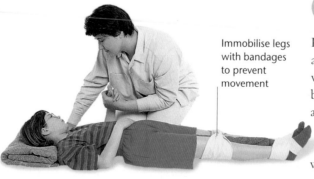

 CALL AN AMBULANCE

Immobilise legs with bandages to prevent movement

Pad between child's legs and immobilise them with a figure-of-eight bandage around feet and ankles and a broad-fold bandage around both knees. Monitor her while you wait, *see p.14.*

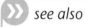
» *see also*
● Severe bleeding, *p.38*
● Shock, *p.36*

Leg injury

Suspect a break if your child is in severe pain. He needs an X-ray or scan to confirm whether or not a bone is broken. Treat the leg in the position found to prevent broken bone ends causing further internal injury.

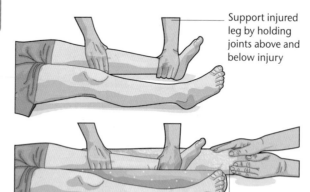

Support injured leg by holding joints above and below injury

Place rolled blankets or towels around injured leg

1 Make your child comfortable and keep him still. Keep his leg in the position you found it by supporting the ankle and knee joints.

2 Support the joints until help arrives. Ask a helper to place padding along the outer side of the limb and between the legs. Cover your child with another blanket to keep him warm. If you suspect shock raise only the *uninjured* leg.

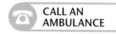 **CALL AN AMBULANCE**

How to splint an injured leg

If you are going to have to wait for help, for example if you are in a remote area, you can splint the injured leg for extra support.

1 Maintain support at the joints. Ask a helper to place padding such as a rolled-up towel or small blanket between the thighs, knees, and ankles. Bring the *uninjured* leg to the broken one.

2 Slide bandages through the hollows under the legs. Place a narrow-fold bandage at the ankle and broad-fold bandages under the knees and below the fracture. Secure the bandage at the ankles first.

3 Secure the broad-fold bandages at the knee then below the injury site – and above if there is room. Tie all knots against the *uninjured* leg.

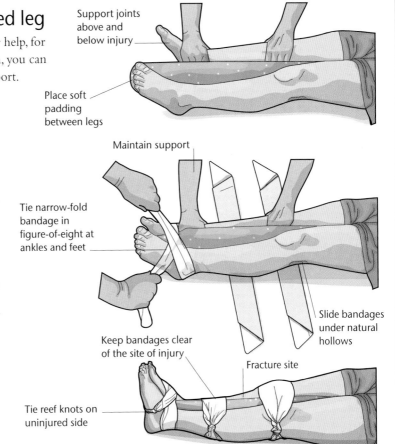

Support joints above and below injury

Place soft padding between legs

Maintain support

Tie narrow-fold bandage in figure-of-eight at ankles and feet

Slide bandages under natural hollows

Keep bandages clear of the site of injury

Fracture site

Tie reef knots on uninjured side

Making broad-fold and narrow-fold bandages

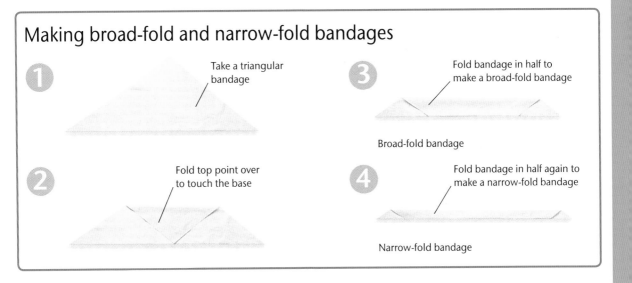

1 Take a triangular bandage

2 Fold top point over to touch the base

3 Fold bandage in half to make a broad-fold bandage

Broad-fold bandage

4 Fold bandage in half again to make a narrow-fold bandage

Narrow-fold bandage

● Follow the RICE procedure:

R Rest the injured part.

I Place a cold pack such as an a bag of **ice** on the injury.

C Provide **comfortable** support.

E Elevate the injured part.

● The child needs to be taken to hospital in the treatment position.

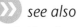 *see also*

● Cold packs, *p.108*

● Leg injury, *p.64*

Knee injury

This type of injury can be very painful, and your child may not be able to move it. The area around the knee joint can swell very quickly.

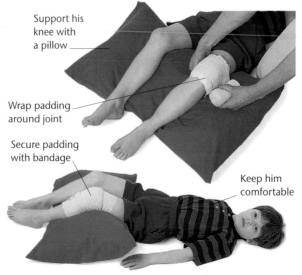

Support his knee with a pillow

Wrap padding around joint

Secure padding with bandage

Keep him comfortable

1 Reassure your child and help him to lie down. Place a pillow under his legs to support them in the most comfortable position. Place a cold pack on the knee. Then wrap a layer of soft padding around it.

2 Secure the padding with a bandage.

☎ **CALL AN AMBULANCE**

 IMPORTANT

● Follow the RICE procedure:

R Rest the injured part.

I Place a cold pack such as a bag of **ice** on the injury.

C Provide **comfortable** support.

E Elevate the injured part.

 see also

● Cold packs, *p.108*

● Leg injury, *p.64*

Foot injury

Your child's foot may be bruised, swollen, and stiff and she may not be able to stand. If caused by crushing, one or more bones may be broken.

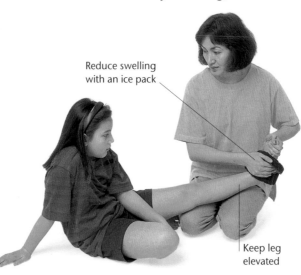

Reduce swelling with an ice pack

Keep leg elevated

1 Sit the child down to rest the injury.

2 Place a cold pack on the injury for 20 minutes then provide comfortable support.

3 Elevate the injury to reduce bruising, pain, and swelling.

▶ **TAKE YOUR CHILD TO HOSPITAL**

Ankle injury

The most common injury is a sprain. Suspect a sprain if your child can't take her full weight on her foot after a fall, or she has twisted, or wrenched, her ankle. She may need an X-ray or scan.

 IMPORTANT

● **If** the pain is very severe or you think a bone could be broken, treat as for a leg injury and TAKE YOUR CHILD to hospital or CALL AN AMBULANCE.

● Follow the RICE procedure:

R Rest the injured part.

I Place a cold pack such as an a bag of **ice** on the injury.

C Provide **comfortable** support.

E Elevate the injured part.

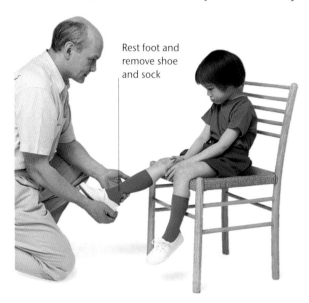

Rest foot and remove shoe and sock

1 Help your child to sit down to rest her foot. Gently remove her sock and shoe before the injured area swells.

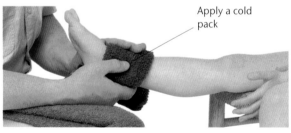

Apply a cold pack

2 Place a cold pack on the injury (*see p.108*) for 20 minutes to minimise swelling.

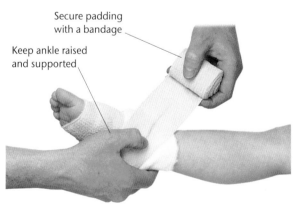

Secure padding with a bandage

Keep ankle raised and supported

3 Provide comfortable support. Wrap a thick layer of soft padding such as cotton wool, around the ankle and secured with a bandage. Make sure the banadge is not too tight.

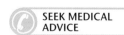 **SEEK MEDICAL ADVICE**

4 Elevate the injury to help reduce bruising, pain, and swelling.

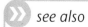 *see also*

● Check circulation, *p.105*

● Cold packs, *p.108*

● Leg injury, *p.64*

Collar bone injury

A collar bone may be broken by indirect force, for example, if a child falls onto her outstretched hand, or by a blow to her shoulder. There will be tenderness in your child's shoulder and arm – increased by attempts to move it – and her head will be turned and inclined to the injured side.

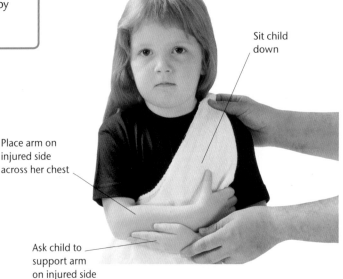

Sit child down

Place arm on injured side across her chest

Ask child to support arm on injured side

1 Help your child to sit down and gently bring the arm on the injured side across her chest. Ask her to support her arm with her hand. Slide a triangular bandage between the child's arm and her chest.

2 Support your child's arm in an arm sling to minimise swelling and discomfort. Make sure the knot is not over the site of injury.

3 For additional support and comfort you can place soft padding between the arm and the sling, then tie a broad-fold bandage around the arm and body.

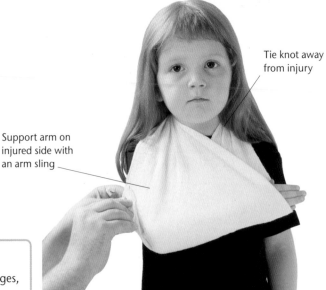

Tie knot away from injury

Support arm on injured side with an arm sling

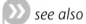

see also
• Triangular bandages, *p.106*

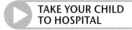

TAKE YOUR CHILD TO HOSPITAL

Rib injury

A child may have a broken rib following a blow to her chest, a heavy fall, or having been crushed. Symptoms include: sharp pain at the fracture site, bruising, swelling, or possible wound on the injured side and pain on breathing.

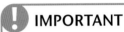

IMPORTANT

● **Do not** give the child anything to eat or drink as an anaesthetic may be needed.

● **If** your child develops breathing difficulties, signs of internal bleeding, or shock, CALL AN AMBULANCE

● **If** your child becomes unresponsive, open airway and check breathing. If breathing place her in the recovery position lying on the injured side to support the chest; if not breathing, begin CPR immediately. CALL AN AMBULANCE

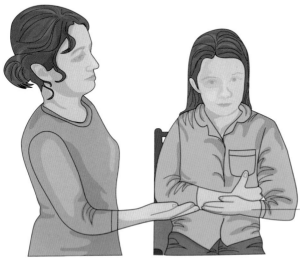

1 Help your child to sit down and gently bring the arm on the injured side across her chest. Ask her to support her arm with her hand; you may need to help her.

Ask child to support arm on injured side

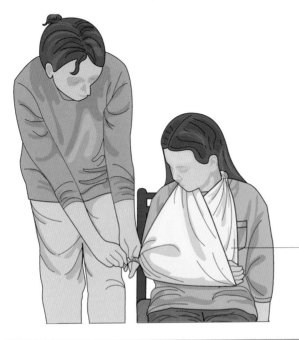

2 Support the arm on the injured side in an arm sling to minimise discomfort.

▶ TAKE YOUR CHILD TO HOSPITAL

Support arm on injured side with a sling

❯❯ see also

● Chest wound, *p.50*

● Internal bleeding, *p.49*

● Shock, *p.36*

● Triangular bandages, *p.106*

● Unresponsive child, *pp.22–27*

Arm injury

The treatment here is for injuries to the upper arm, forearm, and wrist. Move the arm as little as possible to minimise pain.

see also

● Triangular bandages, p.106

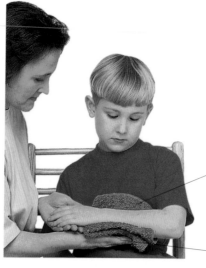

Place padding around injury to protect it

Support injured arm by hand

1 Help your child to sit down. Support the arm and encourage him to help. Place a soft pad around the injury and between his arm and his chest.

2 For extra support place arm in an arm sling; secure the knot on the uninjured side.

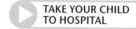
TAKE YOUR CHILD TO HOSPITAL

Elbow injury

Suspect elbow injury if your child is unable to bend her arm; pain is increased by any attempts at movement; there is swelling around the elbow. Keep the injury still as bone ends can damage blood vessels.

see also

● Check circulation, p.105

● Triangular bandages, p.106

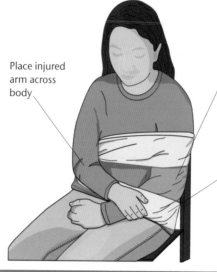

Place injured arm across body

Put soft padding around the joint

Tie broad-fold bandages around arm and body above and below injured elbow

1 Help the child to sit down holding her arm across her body Pad around the injury.

2 Apply broad-fold bandages around the body and arm above and below the elbow. Check circulation at the wrist regularly.

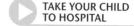
TAKE YOUR CHILD TO HOSPITAL

Hand injury

This type of injury can be very painful. There may be several broken bones, and often a joint is dislocated. If your child's hand was crushed there may also be an open wound.

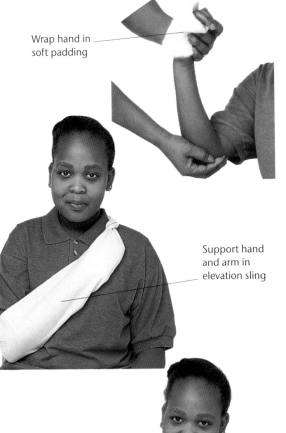

Wrap hand in soft padding

Support hand and arm in elevation sling

Tie broad-fold bandage around arm and body

1 If there is no wound, wrap the injured hand in soft padding. Raise your child's hand into a comfortable position.

2 Place your child's arm in an elevation sling to reduce swelling and provide extra comfort on the journey to hospital.

3 For extra support, tie a broad-fold bandage (*see p.65*) around the arm and body; secure it with a knot on the uninjured side.

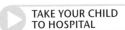

▶ **TAKE YOUR CHILD TO HOSPITAL**

! IMPORTANT

● **If** there is a wound, control the bleeding by pressing a clean dressing or pad over the site of the wound.

Trapped fingers

Hold the fingers under cold running water for a few minutes to relieve the pain and minimise swelling. If the fingers still hurt, apply a cold pack for 10 minutes (*see p.108*).

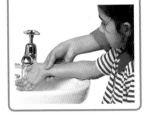

≫ *see also*
● Crush injury, *p.49*
● Finger injury, *p.72*
● Severe bleeding, *p.38*
● Triangular bandages, *p.106*

Finger injury

Injury to a finger is very common in children and can vary from simple
cuts or grazes to broken bones or tendon damage if, for example, the
finger is shut in a door. It is important to get the injury checked as there
are several blood vessels, tendons, and nerves in the finger, which can
be damaged and deformity, bruising, and loss of sensation can result.

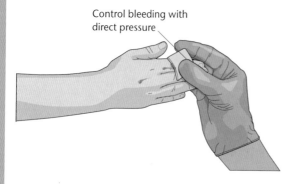

Control bleeding with
direct pressure

1 Apply direct
pressure over a
sterile or clean pad to
control any bleeding; do
not press hard. Stop if this
causes pain as there may
be an underlying fracture.

2 Raise and support
the finger, or ask
your child to hold it up,
to help relieve the pain.

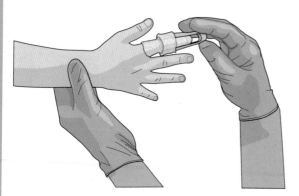

3 Secure the dressing
with a bandage – a
tube gauze bandage is
ideal. For extra comfort
splint the finger to the
next uninjured one.

  **SEEK MEDICAL
ADVICE**

OR

  **TAKE YOUR CHILD
TO HOSPITAL**

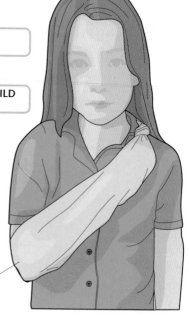

» see also

● Amputation, *p.48*
● Crush injury, *p.49*
● Severe bleeding, *p.38*
● Triangular bandages,
p.106

4 Support the arm
in a raised position
in an elevation sling for
extra comfort on the
journey to hospital.

Apply elevation
sling to help
relieve pain

Cramp

This is a painful muscle spasm that often affects the muscles in the foot, calf, or thigh. Cramp can occur after strenuous exercise or as a result of dehydration through excessive sweating. You can relieve the pain by stretching the affected muscles, then massage them to "relax" the spasm. Give your child water to drink to ease dehydration.

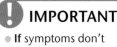

! IMPORTANT
- **If** symptoms don't ease, SEEK MEDICAL ADVICE.

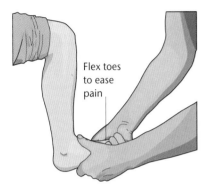

Flex toes to ease pain

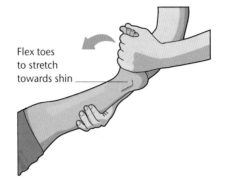

Flex toes to stretch towards shin

For cramp in the foot, encourage your child to stand while you support the affected foot. Flex the toes upwards to stretch the muscles. Once the spasm has passed, massage the underside of the foot with your fingers.

For cramp in the calf muscles, sit or lie the child down and help her straighten her leg while you support her foot. Flex her foot towards her knee to stretch the calf muscles. Once the spasm has passed, massage the back of the leg to relax the muscles.

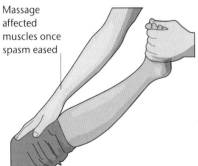

Massage affected muscles once spasm eased

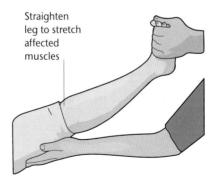

Straighten leg to stretch affected muscles

For cramp in front of thigh, help your child to lie child down, then raise and support her leg. Bend her knee to stretch the muscles. Then, once the spasm has passed, massage the affected muscles.

For cramp in back of thigh, raise and support her leg, and straighten her leg to stretch the muscles. Once the spasm has passed, massage the affected muscles.

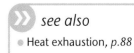

see also
- Heat exhaustion, *p.88*

- **If** your child has injured her arm, support it in a sling.
- **If** bruising is severe or extensive, SEEK MEDICAL ADVICE.

Cold packs

Applying a cold pack to an injury helps minimise swelling and discomfort by reducing blood flow to the area. Make one by filling a plastic bag two-thirds full of ice or use a bag of frozen fruit or vegetables; wrap the bag in a cloth so that the ice does not make direct contact with the skin. You can also use a cloth wrung out in cold water. (*see p.108*).

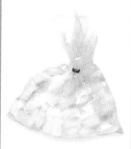

Leave a cold pack in place on an injury for 20 minutes, ideally uncovered.

Bruises and swellings

After a fall or bump, bruising and swelling may develop rapidly. Resting, cooling, and raising the injury will minimise discomfort.

1 Make your child comfortable. Raise and support the injury to rest it and minimise swelling and discomfort.

Raise and support injured part on a pillow

Apply a cold compress to reduce swelling

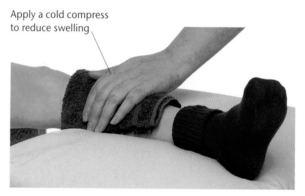

2 To reduce swelling, hold a cold pack against the injury for no more than 20 minutes (*see left*).

Splinter

There is always a risk of infection with splinters. They are often dirty and the bacteria can be carried deep into the skin. Children are most likely to get splinters in their hands and knees as they crawl on the floor.

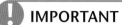

IMPORTANT

● **If** your child is not immunised against tetanus infection, SEEK MEDICAL ADVICE.

● **Do not** poke at the area with a needle to remove the splinter.

● **If** you cannot remove the splinter, or if it breaks off, SEEK MEDICAL ADVICE.

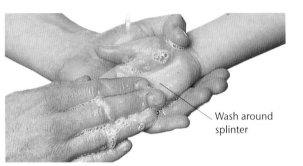

1 Clean the area around the splinter thoroughly with soap and warm water.

Wash around splinter

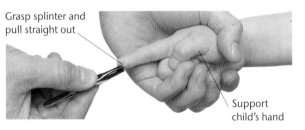

Grasp splinter and pull straight out

Support child's hand

2 Grasp the splinter as close to the skin as possible, and carefully draw it back out at the same angle it went in.

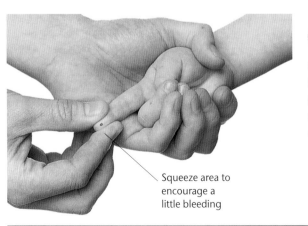

3 Gently squeezing the wound will encourage a little bleeding to flush out dirt. Wash the area again, pat it dry thoroughly, and cover with a plaster.

Squeeze area to encourage a little bleeding

》》 see also

● Infected wound, *p.42*

● Tetanus, *p.42*

! IMPORTANT

● **Do not** touch, or attempt to remove, any foreign object that is sticking to, or embedded in, the eye. TAKE YOUR CHILD TO HOSPITAL.

● **If** eye is still red or sore after the object has been removed, TAKE HER TO HOSPITAL.

For an object that cannot be removed

Tell your child to keep his eyes still, and cover the affected eye with a sterile dressing. Reassure him. TAKE HIM TO HOSPITAL.

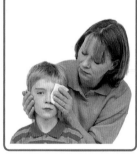

»» see also

● Eye wound, p.44

Object in eye

Tiny hairs or specks of dust on the surface of the eye can be very uncomfortable for a child. However, anything on the surface can generally be washed off easily; try to prevent your child rubbing her eye.

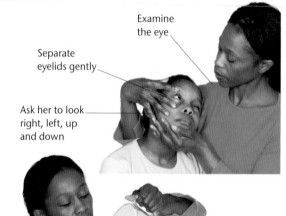

Examine the eye

Separate eyelids gently

Ask her to look right, left, up and down

1 Help your child to sit down, facing the light. Separate the eyelids of the affected eye. Ask her to look right, left, up, and down. Examine her eye thoroughly.

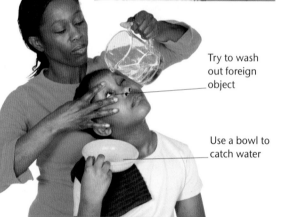

Try to wash out foreign object

Use a bowl to catch water

2 If you can see the foreign object on the surface of the eye, try to rinse it off using a jug of clean water. Tilt her head and aim for the inner corner so that water will wash over her eye. Or, try lifting it off with a damp swab or the corner of a handkerchief.

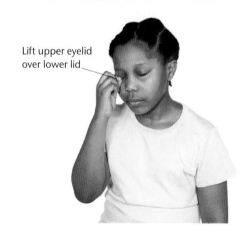

Lift upper eyelid over lower lid

3 If an object is under the eyelid, you can ask an older child to clear it by lifting the upper eyelid over the lower one. You will need to do this for a younger child; if necessary, wrap her in a towel first to stop her grabbing your arms.

Object in ear

Children often push things into their ears. A hard object may become stuck, which can cause pain and temporary deafness; it may even damage the child's ear drum.

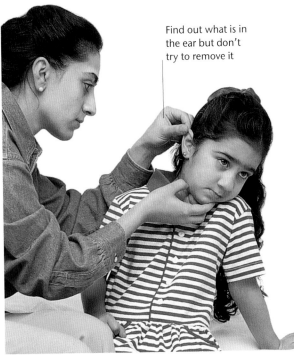

Find out what is in the ear but don't try to remove it

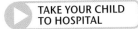

Reassure your child and ask her what she put into her ear. Don't try to remove the object, even if you can see it.

▶ **TAKE YOUR CHILD TO HOSPITAL**

If there is an insect in the ear

If an insect flies or crawls into your child's ear she may be very alarmed.

1 Help her to sit her down. Support her head with the affected ear uppermost.

2 Gently flood the ear with tepid water so that the insect floats out.

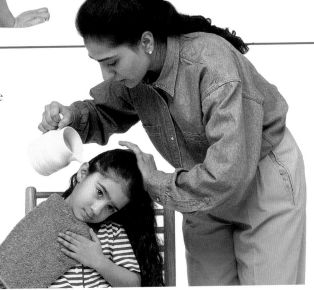

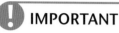
Object in nose

If your child has something stuck in his nose his breathing may be difficult or noisy and his nose may be swollen. Smelly or blood-stained discharge from the nose indicates an object has been present for a while.

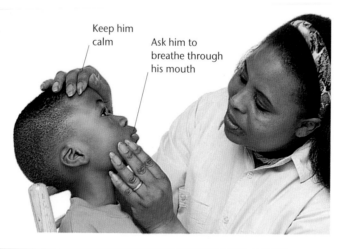

Keep him calm

Ask him to breathe through his mouth

1 Reassure your child and try to find out what he put in his nose. Tell him not to touch it.

2 Tell your child to breathe through his mouth.

> ▶ **TAKE YOUR CHILD TO HOSPITAL**

Swallowed object

Young children often put small objects in their mouths and may swallow them. Most objects will pass straight through the digestive system. Small button batteries are dangerous as they contain corrosive chemicals.

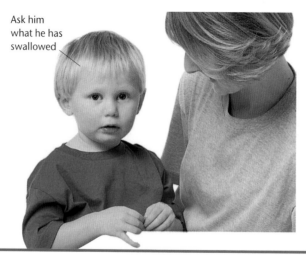

Ask him what he has swallowed

1 Reassure your child. Try to find out what he child has swallowed.

2 If the object is small and smooth like a pebble or a coin, there is little danger.

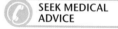

> **SEEK MEDICAL ADVICE**

Animal and human bites

The main risk with any bite is infection; sharp pointed teeth can carry germs deep into the skin. Severe wounds with torn edges may need stitches. There is a risk of rabies from animals from outside the UK.

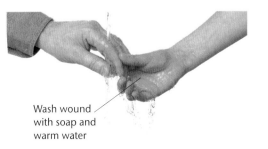

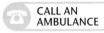
Wash wound with soap and warm water

1 Wash the wound thoroughly, using soap and warm water. Rinse the wound under cold running water for at least five minutes to wash away any dirt.

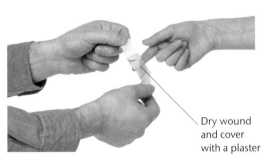

Dry wound and cover with a plaster

2 Gently, but thoroughly, pat the wound dry with a clean pad or tissue. Cover it with a plaster or a small sterile dressing.

SEEK MEDICAL ADVICE

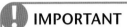
! IMPORTANT

● **If** the bleeding is severe, treat your child for shock.

● **If** your child is bitten by an animal while you are abroad, you must take your child to hospital for advice about rabies.

● **Make** sure child's tetanus immunisation is up to date.

》 see also
● Infected wound, *p.42*
● Severe bleeding, *p.38*
● Shock, *p.36*

For a serious animal bite

1 If bleeding is severe, apply direct pressure over the wound, preferably over a sterile dressing or clean non-fluffy pad. Ask a helper to

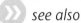
CALL AN AMBULANCE

2 Cover the wound with a sterile dressing or pad and bandage firmly in place to help maintain direct pressure; make sure the bandage is not too tight, (*see p. 105*). Treat child for shock if necessary. Monitor the child's breathing, pulse, and level of reponse while waiting for help to arrive.

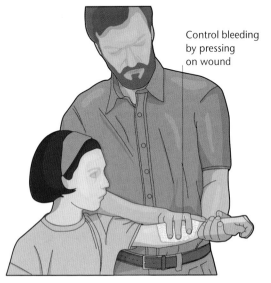
Control bleeding by pressing on wound

Insect sting

Bee, wasp, or hornet stings can be very alarming for a child, but they are rarely dangerous. Your child will experience a sharp pain followed by soreness, red skin, and slight swelling around the site of the sting.

If sting is in mouth

Give your child an ice cube to suck or cold water to sip and SEEK MEDICAL ADVICE. If swelling develops, CALL AN AMBULANCE.

see also
● Anaphylactic shock, p.91

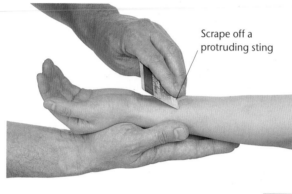

Scrape off a protruding sting

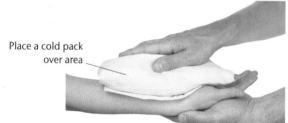

Place a cold pack over area

① If the sting is still in the skin, brush or scrape it off sideways with your fingernail or a plastic card. Don't try to remove it with tweezers as you may inject more poison into your child.

② Place a cold pack (see p.108) on the site for about 20 minutes to minimise the pain and swelling. Rest the injured part and if pain and swelling persists,

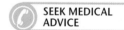
SEEK MEDICAL ADVICE

Nettle rash

If your child brushes against nettles he will have a blotchy, red, itchy rash that may frighten him. Reassure him and soothe the rash.

❗ IMPORTANT
● If the rash is extensive, SEEK MEDICAL ADVICE.

see also
● Allergy, p.90
● Cold pack, p.108

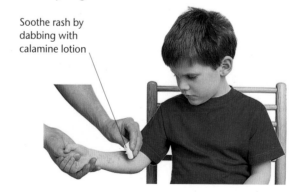

Soothe rash by dabbing with calamine lotion

① To relieve the itching, dab the rash with cotton wool soaked in calamine lotion.

② Alternatively, place a cold pack over the rash until the pain is relieved, about 20 minutes.

Tick bite

Found in woodland and long grass, ticks are minute, spider-like creatures that carry viruses and bacteria, including Borrelia, which cause Lyme disease. They attach themselves to people and animals to suck blood and can swell up to the size of a pea. Always check yourself and your child after walking in areas where ticks are likely to be found.

1 Using fine-toothed tweezers, grasp the tick as close to the child's skin as possible. Pull the tick's "head" upwards using steady pressure. Don't twist or crush the tick as this can leave mouth parts (and saliva) embedded in the child.

Grasp head as close to skin as possible

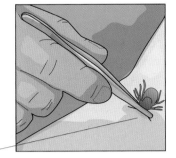

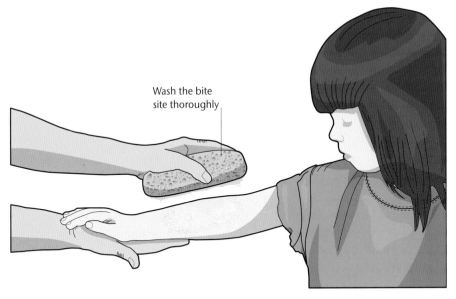

Wash the bite site thoroughly

2 Wash the area around the bite with soap and water.

SEEK MEDICAL ADVICE

3 Put the tick into a sealed plastic bag and take it to your doctor as he or she may want to check that it is complete as well as for the bacteria that cause Lyme disease.

4 If your child develops a rash around the bite site or she starts to display any flu-like symptoms, *see box right*, seek urgent medical advice.

! IMPORTANT

● **Do not** attempt to burn the tick or cover it with petroleum jelly in your attempt to remove it. You could injure the child and it may cause the tick to regurgitate infective fluid into her.

● **If** you can't remove the tick or you think mouth parts remain SEEK URGENT MEDICAL ADVICE.

Lyme disease

The first sign of this may be a circular rash at the site of the bite that can develop up to 30 days later. The rash is described as looking like the bull's eye on a dart board. There may also be flu-like symptoms and if left untreated symptoms affecting joints, heart, and nervous system can develop weeks or months later.

» see also
● Fever p.94

» *see also*

• Anaphylactic shock, p.91

• Checking vital signs, p.14

Jellyfish sting

Jellyfish venom is contained in stinging cells that stick to a child's skin. Stings from marine creatures in temperate waters may not be dangerous, but those in tropical waters can cause severe poisoning.

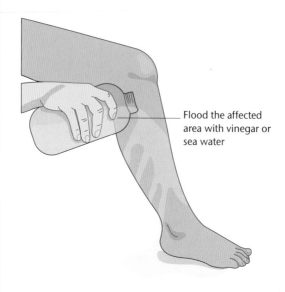

Flood the affected area with vinegar or sea water

1 Pour vinegar if available or sea water over the affected area to incapacitate the stinging cells.

2 Help the child to sit down and immobilise the area as for snake bite, opposite.

☎ **CALL AN AMBULANCE**

3 Monitor breathing, pulse, and level of response while you wait.

Marine puncture wound

When trodden on, the spines from marine creatures such as weever fish can puncture the skin, causing painful swelling and soreness. The spines can also break off and become embedded in a child's foot.

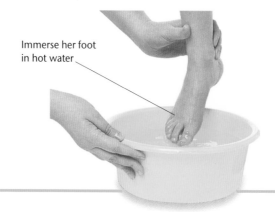

Immerse her foot in hot water

Immerse the injury in water as hot as your child can bear for about 30 minutes. Top up as the water cools, but be careful not to scald her.

▶ **TAKE YOUR CHILD TO HOSPITAL**

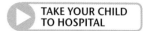

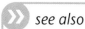

Snake bite

If your child is bitten by a snake there will be two puncture marks. There may also be redness at the site and he may be feeling sick or vomiting, and be sweating. There may be disturbed vision and difficulty breathing.

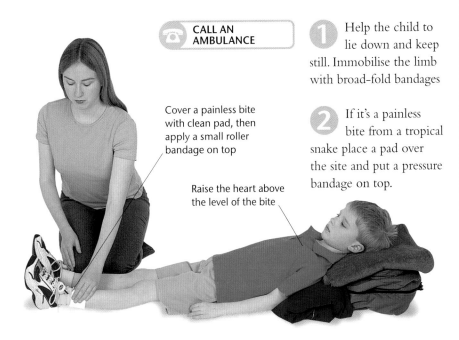

☎ CALL AN AMBULANCE

Cover a painless bite with clean pad, then apply a small roller bandage on top

Raise the heart above the level of the bite

1 Help the child to lie down and keep still. Immobilise the limb with broad-fold bandages

2 If it's a painless bite from a tropical snake place a pad over the site and put a pressure bandage on top.

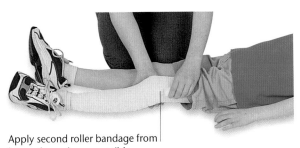

Apply second roller bandage from bite as far up leg as possible

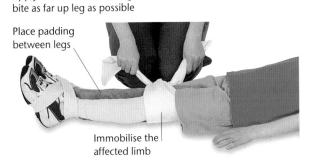

Place padding between legs

Immobilise the affected limb

3 Apply a second pressure bandage that extends from the bite as far up the limb as possible. Check circulation after bandaging (*see p. 105*), and loosen if necessary.

4 Immobilise the limb with folded triangular bandages and padding (or a sling if it's on the arm). Monitor breathing, pulse, and level of response while you wait for help.

» *see also*

- Anaphylactic shock, *p.91*
- Checking vital signs, *p.14*
- Triangular bandages, *p.65 and p.106*
- Unresponsive baby, *pp.19–21*
- Unresponsive child, *p.22–27*

Hypothermia

This develops if the body temperature falls below 35°C (95°F) and if it falls further it is very serious. An older child is most likely to develop it outside in poor weather conditions, especially if there is a high wind-chill factor, or if a child falls into cold water. For babies, *see opposite*. Your child is suffering from hypothermia if she is shivering, has cold pale skin, is listless or confused, is becoming unresponsive, and she has slow breathing and a weakening pulse.

For a child outside

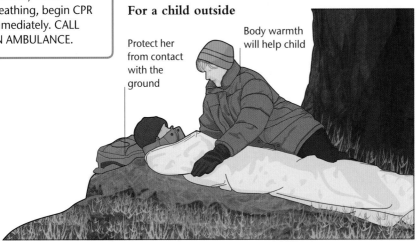

Protect her from contact with the ground

Body warmth will help child

Take your child to a shelter. If there isn't one nearby lay her on a layer of dry insulating material such as heather or bracken and protect her from the wind. Wrap her in a dry sleeping bag and a foil blanket if available. Use your body to keep her warm too.

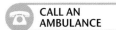
☎ CALL AN AMBULANCE

For a child indoors

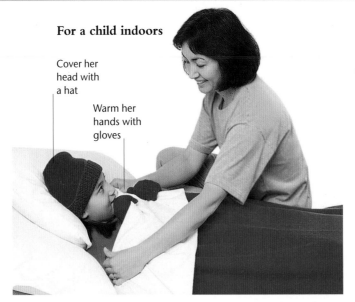

Cover her head with a hat

Warm her hands with gloves

1 If you can get to a shelter or your child is indoors, remove any wet clothes and replace them with dry ones. Cover her with plenty of blankets – you can put her in bed. Cover her head with a hat and make sure that the room is warm. Stay with her.

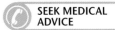
SEEK MEDICAL ADVICE

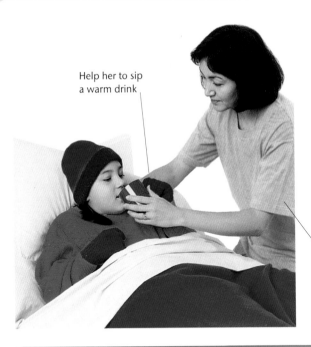

Help her to sip
a warm drink

2 Give your child a warm drink and some high-energy foods, such as chocolate. Monitor her breathing, pulse, temperature, and level of response. Do not leave her alone until you are sure that her temperature has returned to normal.

Stay with her until
her temperature has
returned to normal

>> see also

● Checking vital signs,
p.14

● Unresponsive baby,
pp.19–21

● Unresponsive child,
p.22–27

Hypothermia in babies

A baby's temperature regulation is not fully developed. He can lose body heat rapidly and develop hypothermia in a cold room. Suspect hypothermia if: your baby's skin feels cold; he is limp and unusually quiet; and he refuses to feed.

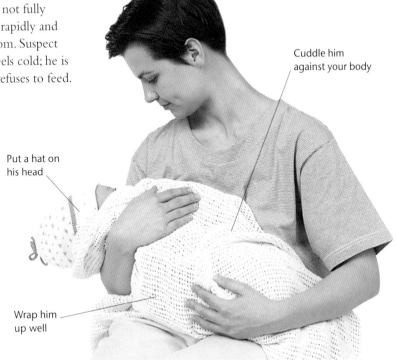

Cuddle him
against your body

Put a hat on
his head

Wrap him
up well

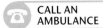
**CALL AN
AMBULANCE**

1 Re-warm a baby by warming the room or taking him to a warm room. Wrap him in blankets.

2 Put a hat on his head and cuddle him against your body so that he is warmed by your body heat.

Frostbite

If the skin is broken

If there are any open wounds or the frozen skin is broken, cover the area with a soft gauze dressing and bandage it lightly in place. TAKE YOUR CHILD TO HOSPITAL.

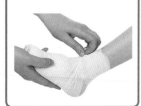

If children are exposed to extreme weather conditions, the tissues of the fingers and toes may freeze. Your child may have frostbite if she has pins and needles in her fingers or toes with numbness and hard, stiff skin that is turning white and waxy. Shelter your child before treating her.

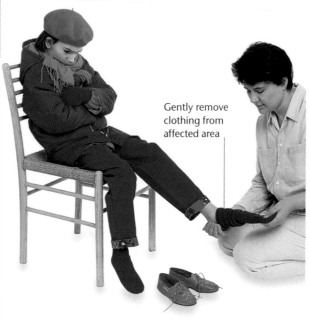

Gently remove clothing from affected area

1 While you are still outside, advise your child to put her hands under her armpits to use her body warmth to prevent the condition worsening.

2 Once in a warm shelter, help her to sit down then start treatment. Gently remove constrictions from the affected area such as shoes, socks, and/or gloves and rings. Undo her coat. Start warming the affected area with your hands, in your lap, and/or in the child's armpits; don't rub them.

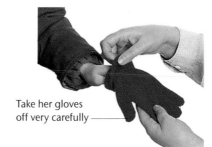

Take her gloves off very carefully

3 Place the affected part(s) in warm water – it should be around 40°C (104°F). Pat dry and cover with a light gauze bandage.

4 Raise the affected area to reduce swelling. Give your child the recommended dose of paracetamol (not aspirin) to ease the pain.

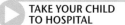

▶ **TAKE YOUR CHILD TO HOSPITAL**

Sunburn

Sunburn is red, itchy, and tender. Babies and young children are very vulnerable: keep them in shade; apply sun block; put on a hat and cover with protective clothing in hot weather.

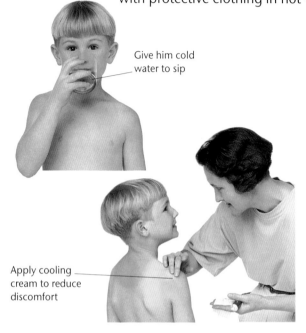

Give him cold water to sip

Apply cooling cream to reduce discomfort

1 Move your child into the shade or into a cool room and give him a cold drink. Cool the skin by dabbing it with cold water.

2 Apply calamine lotion or an after-sun cream to soothe the skin. Make sure it is a cream that you *know* your child is not allergic to.

> **IMPORTANT**
> - If there is blistering, or other skin damage SEEK MEDICAL ADVICE.
> - If your child is restless, flushed, dizzy, or has a temperature or headache, he may have heatstroke.

>> *see also*
> - Heat exhaustion, *p.88*
> - Heatstroke, *p.89*

Heat rash

This a prickly, red rash that develops particularly around the sweat glands on the chest and back and under the arms.

1 Help your child to sit down in a cool room and undress her. Sponge the affected area with cool water.

2 Pat her almost dry with a soft towel, leaving the skin slightly damp. Apply calamine lotion to the rash.

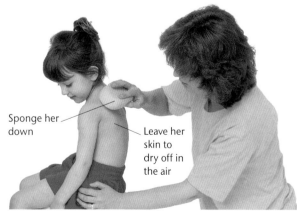

Sponge her down

Leave her skin to dry off in the air

> **IMPORTANT**
> - If your baby develops heat rash, remove some of her clothes to cool her, or bathe her in tepid water. Dry her gently, leaving her skin slightly damp.
> - If the rash has not faded after 12 hours, or if she develops a raised temperature, SEEK MEDICAL ADVICE.

>> *see also*
> - Heat exhaustion, *p.88*

Heat exhaustion

This is caused by a loss of water and salts from the body because of excessive sweating. Children who are not used to the heat are most at risk especially if unwell, particularly if they have diarrhoea and vomiting. Suspect this if a child: complains of a headache, dizziness and nausea; is sweating; has pale, clammy skin; cramps; and a rapid, weakening pulse.

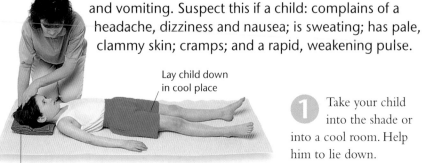

Lay child down in cool place

Put folded towel or cushion under head

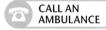 **1** Take your child into the shade or into a cool room. Help him to lie down.

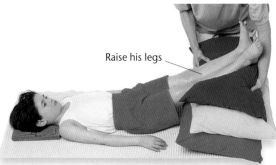

Raise his legs

2 Raise and support your child's legs on some pillows. This improves blood supply to the brain. Encourage him to rest quietly.

3 Help your child to sip as much cool water as he can manage. Later give oral rehydration salts or an isotonic drink to replace salt lost from the body.

 SEEK MEDICAL ADVICE

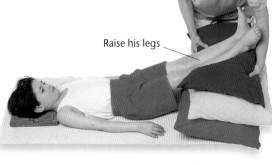

Give him as much cool water as he can manage

4 Monitor breathing, pulse, level of response, and temperature. If his condition worsens,

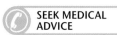 **CALL AN AMBULANCE**

⟫ see also

● Checking vital signs, *p.14*

● Heatstroke, *opposite*

● Unresponsive baby, *pp.19–21*

● Unresponsive child, *p.22–27*

Heatstroke

This is a serious condition that develops if the body becomes overheated in hot surroundings, because the "thermostsat" that controls body temperature fails so the body cannot cool itself. Treat your child for heatstroke if she: develops a sudden headache; is confused; has hot, flushed, dry skin; has a full bounding pulse; is becoming unresponsive; has a temperature of over 40°C (104°F).

! IMPORTANT

● **If** a baby or very young child develops heatstroke, undress him completely in a cool room.

● **If** your child becomes unresponsive, open his airway and check breathing. If breathing, place in the recovery position; if not breathing, begin CPR immediately.

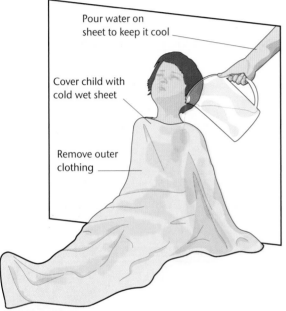

Pour water on sheet to keep it cool

Cover child with cold wet sheet

Remove outer clothing

1 Quickly move child into a cool place. Remove as much outer clothing as you can.

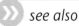 **CALL AN AMBULANCE**

2 Help the child to sit down on the ground. Support her with cushions and/or against a wall and wrap her in a cold, wet sheet. Gently pour more water over the sheet to keep it cool.

3 Leave the sheet over the child until her temperature falls to 38°C (100.4°F) under the tongue or 37.5°C (99.5°F) under the armpit.

4 Replace wet sheet with a dry, light cover. Reassure your child and monitor breathing, pulse, level of response, and temperature while waiting for help to arrive. Repeat the cooling if her temperature starts to rise again.

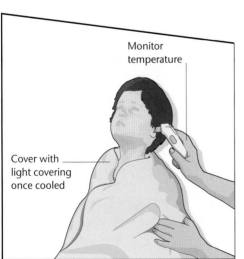

Monitor temperature

Cover with light covering once cooled

» see also

● Checking vital signs, *p.14*

● Unresponsive baby, *pp.19–21*

● Unresponsive child, *p.22–27*

! IMPORTANT

● If the child's condition does not improve, the rash worsens, or he develops breathing difficulties and/or swelling of the face or neck, or is becoming distressed, treat for anaphylactic shock, *opposite*. CALL AN AMBULANCE.

Allergy

This is an abnormal reaction in the body's defences in response to exposure to an allergen and symptoms vary depending on the cause. Common allergens include pollen, dust, some foods such as nuts, shellfish and eggs, as well as insect stings or bites. Mild allergy normally develops slowly and a child may have an itchy rash or raised blotchy areas on her skin, possible swelling of the feet, hands and/or face, sneezing, red itchy eyes, wheezing, even tummy pain, vomiting, and diarrhoea – any of which can be very uncomfortable.

1 Try to identify the cause and try to remove the allergen from the child or the child from allergen. If pollen is the allergen, move him indoors. If he has a reaction to washing powder, remove the affected clothing.

2 Treat any symptoms. For example, soothe an itchy rash with calamine lotion. Suggest he uses his asthma medication if necessary.

3 Talk to your pharmacist as some mild allergies can be controlled with over-the-counter medication formulated for children. If the symptoms persist,

SEEK MEDICAL ADVICE

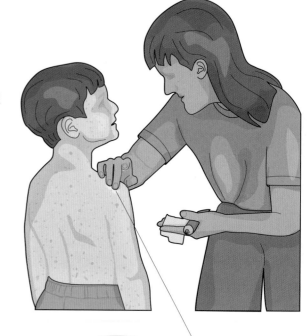

Dab calamine on itchy skin

Offer recommended dose of antihistamine medication

» see also

● Asthma, *p.35*

● Anaphylactic shock, *opposite*

Anaphylactic shock

This is a severe allergic reaction affecting the whole body that may develop within a few minutes of, for example, the injection of a drug, an insect sting, or ingestion of a food. It causes constriction of the air passages and swelling of the face and neck that can result in suffocation. Suspect anaphylactic shock if alongside symptoms of mild allergy, your child has increased difficulty breathing. Skin may be blotchy or flushed.

! IMPORTANT

• If child has a known allergy and has her own medication help her to use it or give it to her yourself, *see below*.

• If your child becomes unresponsive, open her airway and check breathing. If breathing, place in the recovery position; if not breathing, begin CPR immediately.

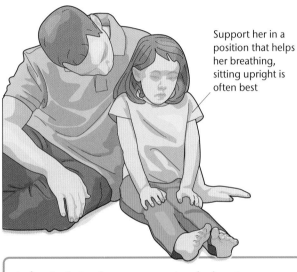

Support her in a position that helps her breathing, sitting upright is often best

☎ CALL AN AMBULANCE

1 Help your child into a position that helps breathing. Help her with her medication.

2 Monitor breathing, pulse, and level of response while you wait for the ambulance. If pulse weakens and she becomes pale, treat for shock.

» see also

• Checking vital signs, *p.14*

• Shock, *p.36*

• Unresponsive baby, *pp.19–21*

• Unresponsive child, *pp.22–27*

Administering an auto-injector

A child with a known allergy is often prescribed medication – usually an auto-injector of adrenaline – to use in the event of a reaction.

1 Hold the injector with your fist and remove the safety cap; don't put your thumb over the end.

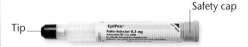

Tip

Safety cap

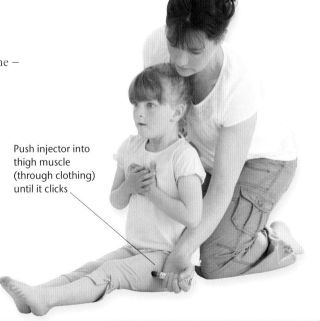

Push injector into thigh muscle (through clothing) until it clicks

2 Place the tip firmly against the child's thigh to release the medication. Hold it in place for 10 seconds, remove it and rub the injection site for 10 seconds; repeat at 5-minute intervals if there's no improvement.

Diabetic emergency

If a child with Type 1 diabetes has low blood sugar he will be: weak or hungry; confused or behave aggressively; sweating; very pale. He may also have a strong, bounding pulse and breathing may be shallow.

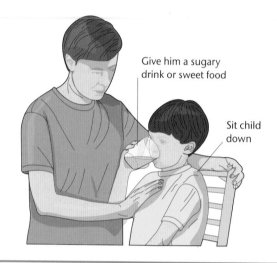

Give him a sugary drink or sweet food

Sit child down

Help your child to sit down and give him 15–20g of glucose (150ml orange juice, 3tsp sugar, or 3 jelly babies) to raise blood sugar levels. If he recovers give him more. Check his glucose levels and monitor him until he is fully recovered.

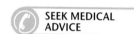

SEEK MEDICAL ADVICE

If the child becomes unresponsive

If a child with diabetes is unresponsive, **do not** offer her anything to eat or drink.

☎ **CALL AN AMBULANCE**

1 Open the airway and check breathing, *see p.22.*

2 If she is breathing, place her in the recovery position, *see p.26.*

3 If she is not breathing, begin CPR straightaway, *see p.24.*

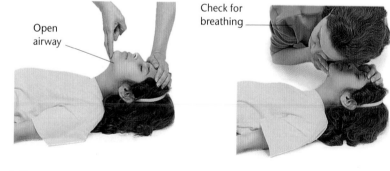

Open airway

Check for breathing

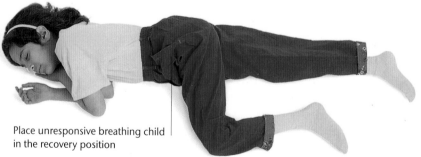

Place unresponsive breathing child in the recovery position

Faint

Your child may be about to faint if she complains of feeling weak, giddy and sick, and is very pale. The period of unresponsiveness is brief and accompanied by a slow pulse; recovery is rapid and complete.

1 Help your child to lie down and raise her legs above the level of her heart; this helps improve the blood flow to the vital organs. Support her legs on a pile of cushions or folded blankets.

2 Reassure your child and help her to sit her up gradually. If she starts to feel faint again help her to lie back down until she feels better, then try again. If you are concerned about your child after the faint,

SEEK MEDICAL ADVICE

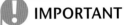

! IMPORTANT

● **Do not** sit your child on a chair with her head down if she is feeling faint as she may fall off and hurt herself.

● **If** your child becomes unresponsive, open her airway and check breathing. If breathing, place in the recovery position; if not breathing, begin CPR immediately. CALL AN AMBULANCE.

» see also

● Unresponsive child, pp.22–27

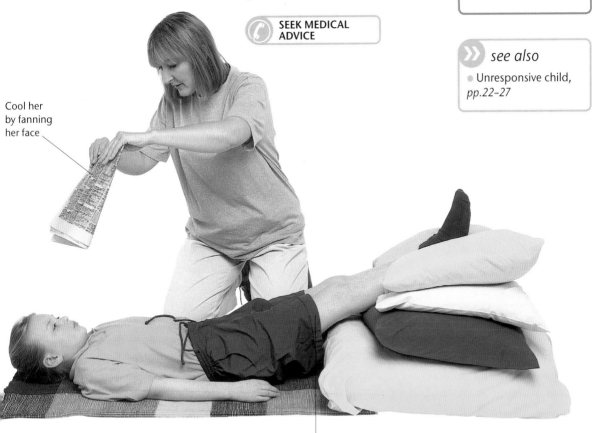

Cool her by fanning her face

Raise her legs above the level of her heart

! IMPORTANT

● **If** your baby is under three months old, you should not give her paracetamol syrup, unless you are advised to do so by your doctor.

● **If** your child is very hot, take as many clothes off as possible; do not sponge with water to cool her.

● **If** your child complains of a severe headache, suspect meningitis. TAKE YOUR CHILD TO HOSPITAL or CALL AN AMBULANCE.

● **Raised** body temperature can be caused by overheating, *see* Heatstroke *p.88*.

Fever

A body temperature that is above 37°C (98.6°F) indicates fever. An infection is the usual cause. A moderate fever is not harmful, but a temperature above 39°C (102.2°F) can be dangerous and may trigger seizures, particularly in very young children. Your child has a fever if she: has a raised temperature; looks very pale; complains she feels cold with goose pimples; is shivering, with chattering teeth. As the fever advances she will have hot, flushed skin, be sweating, and have a headache.

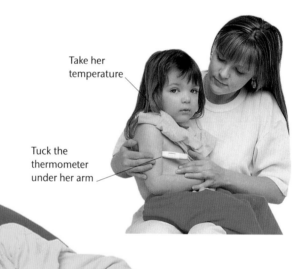

Take her temperature

Tuck the thermometer under her arm

Leave a drink beside her

Give her the recommended dose of paracetamol syrup

1 Take your child's temperature. If you are using a digital thermometer, on a young child lift your child's arm and tuck the pointed end into her armpit. Lower her arm over it and against her side and leave the thermometer in place until it beeps; an under arm reading will be 0.5°C (1°F) lower than under the tongue.

2 Make your child comfortable on a bed or sofa, but do not cover her. To help bring down her temperature, make sure she has plenty of water or diluted fruit juice to drink.

3 You can give her the recommended dose of paracetamol syrup (not aspirin) to help reduce her temperature; never give aspirin to anyone under the age of 16 years.

►► see also

● Febrile seizures, *p.96*
● Heatstroke, *p.88*
● Meningitis, *opposite*

Meningitis

This is a life-threatening infection affecting the tissues that surround the brain. In the early stages your child will have a flu-like illness with a high temperature. He may tell you he has cold hands and feet, joint and limb pain, and he may have mottled or very pale skin. As infection develops he is likely to have a headache, neck stiffness, and begin vomiting. His eyes may be sensitive to light and he will become increasingly drowsy. Later, a red or purple rash may develop that does not disappear if pressed.

> ## ❗ IMPORTANT
>
> ● **If** there is any delay contacting medical advice, or if you are concerned about your child's condition, TAKE YOUR CHILD TO HOSPITAL or CALL AN AMBULANCE even if you have already seen a doctor.
>
> ● **In** some cases, the rash may not develop, or if it does, it will be one of the last symptoms to appear.

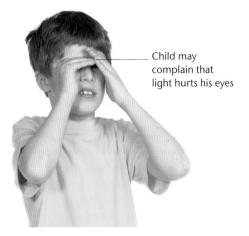

Child may complain that light hurts his eyes

1 If your child has a high fever and a flu-like illness, monitor him carefully. If light hurts his eyes, let him rest in a darker room and monitor for other signs. Treat fever. Give him plenty of fluids to drink and the recommended dose of paracetamol syrup (not aspirin).

☎ SEEK MEDICAL ADVICE

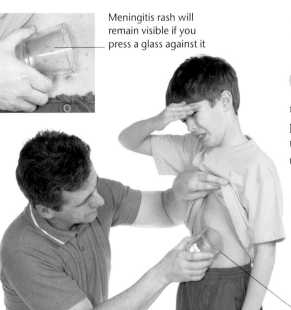

Meningitis rash will remain visible if you press a glass against it

2 Check your child's body for signs of a rash. If you see any spots, press a glass gently against them. If you can still see the spots through the glass.

☎ CALL AN AMBULANCE

Press side of a glass against the rash

> **»** *see also*
> ● Febrile seizures, *p.96*
> ● Fever, *opposite*

! IMPORTANT

● **Do not** sponge a child with tepid water to cool her as there is a risk of overcooling her.

● **If** a child becomes unresponsive, open her airway and check breathing. If breathing, place in the recovery position; if she is not breathing, begin CPR immediately. CALL AN AMBULANCE.

Febrile seizures

Young children may develop these seizures when they have a high temperature. Suspect a febrile seizure if: your child is flushed and sweating with a very hot forehead; her eyes are rolled upwards, and possibly fixed or squinting; she is holding her breath and her face looks blue; she is shaking vigorously, arches her back and clenches her fists.

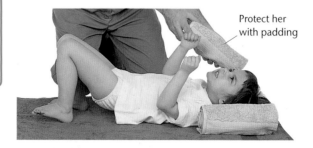

Protect her with padding

1 Place soft padding, such as towels or pillows, around your child so that even violent movement will not lead to injury.

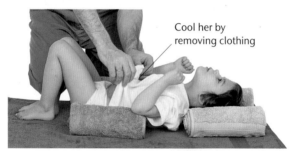

Cool her by removing clothing

2 Undress your child to help cool her down. Make sure there is a good supply of cool fresh air, but be careful not to overcool her.

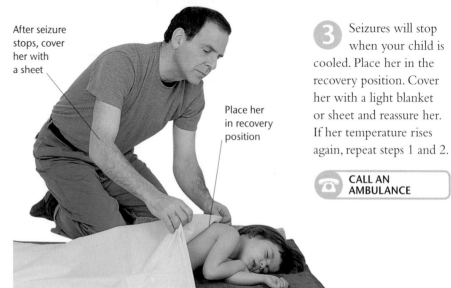

After seizure stops, cover her with a sheet

Place her in recovery position

3 Seizures will stop when your child is cooled. Place her in the recovery position. Cover her with a light blanket or sheet and reassure her. If her temperature rises again, repeat steps 1 and 2.

☎ CALL AN AMBULANCE

» see also

● Fever, p.94

● Unresponsive baby, pp.19–21

● Unresponsive child, pp.22–27

Epileptic seizures

These are caused by a disturbance in the electrical activity of the brain. A seizure may progress through stages: sudden loss of responsiveness, sometimes with a cry; rigidity and arching of back; breathing may cease; jerking or vigorous shaking movements begin; froth or bubbles appear at the mouth, possibly blood stained; loss of bladder or bowel control. The child will be responsive again within a few minutes and appear dazed. Afterwards she may fall into a deep sleep.

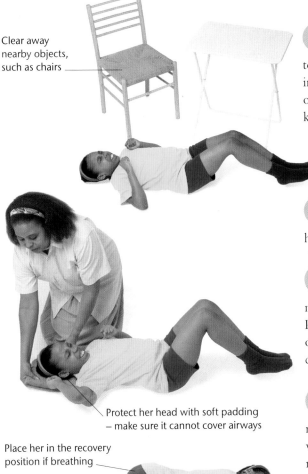

Clear away nearby objects, such as chairs

Protect her head with soft padding – make sure it cannot cover airways

Place her in the recovery position if breathing

1 If your child starts to fall, help her to the floor. Prevent injury by clearing away objects that she may knock against.

2 Place padding under or around her head to prevent injury.

3 When her seizure is over, your child may become unresponsive. Remove any padding and open her airway and check breathing.

4 If she is breathing, place her in the recovery position. Stay with her until she is fully recovered. She may feel dazed and behave oddly, or sleep deeply.

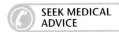 **SEEK MEDICAL ADVICE**

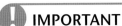 **IMPORTANT**

- **Do not** hold her down or try to move her during the seizure.

- **Do not** put anything in her mouth or give her anything to eat or drink.

- **Look** for a card or bracelet alerting you to the fact that a child has a history of epilepsy.

- **If** your child has never had a seizure before, a seizure lasts more than 5 minutes, if she has repeated seizures, or if she is unresponsive for more than 10 minutes CALL AN AMBULANCE.

Absence seizures

These seizures can be recognised by a momentary "switching off", some facial twitching, or distracted movements such as lip-smacking. If this happens, reassure the child and SEEK MEDICAL ADVICE.

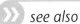 *see also*

- Unresponsive baby, *pp.19–21*

- Unresponsive child, *pp.22–27*

Vomiting and diarrhoea

A baby or child who is suffering repeated vomiting and/or diarrhoea can become dehydrated very quickly. It is important to replace lost fluids by giving your child sips of cooled, boiled water. Don't give a baby or child milk unless you are breastfeeding.

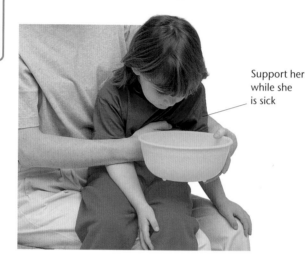

Support her while she is sick

1 If your child is being sick, hold her over a bowl. Support her upper body with your free hand while she is being sick. Reassure her.

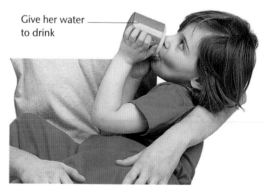

Give her water to drink

2 Give her drinks of water to replace any fluid loss and to remove the unpleasant taste. Encourage her to sip each drink slowly.

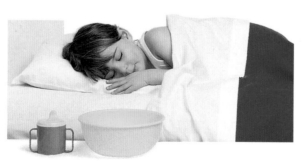

3 Let her rest quietly, in bed if she wants to. Make sure the bowl is still at hand in case she is sick again, and give a fresh drink of water. When she is hungry again offer easily digested foods such as pasta, bread, or potatoes in the first 24 hours.

Stomachache

This is generally caused by a stomach upset as a result of an infection such as food poisoning.

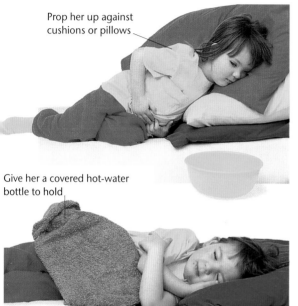

Prop her up against cushions or pillows

Give her a covered hot-water bottle to hold

1 Make your child comfortable on a sofa or bed. Help her to lie back against cushions or pillows. She may want to be sick so leave a container near her.

2 Warmth may help to relieve the pain. Fill a hot-water bottle – it must be covered – and give it to your child to hold against her stomach. Avoid giving her anything to eat until pain subsides.

! IMPORTANT

- If the pain is severe, or does not subside after 30 minutes and/or is accompanied by fever and vomiting, TAKE YOUR CHILD TO HOSPITAL or CALL AN AMBULANCE.

- If your child has been "winded", sit her down and loosen clothing around her waist. The pain should ease quickly. If in you are in any doubt, SEEK MEDICAL ADVICE.

Appendicitis

Suspect appendicitis if your child complains of waves of pain in the middle of his abdomen or of acute pain settling in the right lower abdomen. He may also have a raised temperature, no appetite, nausea, vomiting, and diarrhoea.

Suspected appendicitis must be treated promptly. Help your child to lie down. Do not give him anything to eat or drink as he may need an anaesthetic.

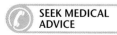

SEEK MEDICAL ADVICE

Pain may start here

Pain settles here

Pressure-change earache

This may happen on plane journeys, particularly when taking off or landing, or when travelling through tunnels. To make the ears "pop" so that the pressure is relieved, an older child should close her mouth, hold her nose and blow down it. Sucking a sweet may also help.

Earache

This is most commonly caused by an ear infection following a cold or flu. Earache can be the result of a child putting something in her ear.

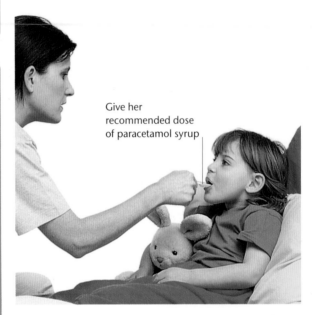

Give her recommended dose of paracetamol syrup

1 Make your child comfortable. Help her to sit up supported by pillows or cushions if lying down makes the earache worse. You can give the recommended dose of paracetamol syrup (not aspirin). Never give asprin to anyone under the age of 16 years.

2 Applying heat may help to soothe the pain. Prepare a covered hot-water bottle and tell your child to lie down with her painful ear against it.

Provide a covered hot-water bottle to place against her ear

Prop her up with pillows

Toothache

A toddler who complains of toothache may have a new tooth coming through. An older child may have tooth decay or an infection.

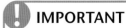

IMPORTANT

- **If** jaw is swollen and pain is severe, SEEK DENTAL ADVICE.

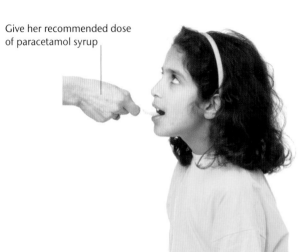

Give her recommended dose of paracetamol syrup

1 Give your child the recommended dose of paracetamol syrup (not aspirin) to relieve the pain. Never give asprin to anyone under the age of 16 years. Arrange an early appointment with your child's dentist if pain persists.

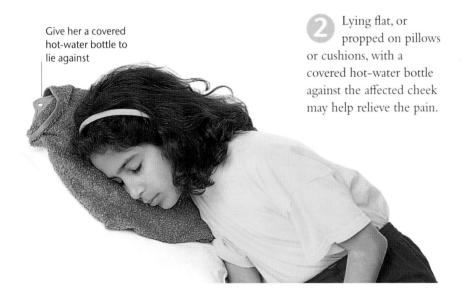

Give her a covered hot-water bottle to lie against

2 Lying flat, or propped on pillows or cushions, with a covered hot–water bottle against the affected cheek may help relieve the pain.

First aid kit

A well-stocked first aid kit

- Disposable gloves (choose latex free)
- Small and large roller bandages
- Tube-gauze bandage
- Blunt-ended scissors
- Plastic tweezers
- Pack of gauze swabs
- Triangular bandages
- Tape for securing dressing pads and bandages – ideally hypoallergenic
- Sterile non-adhesive pads
- Waterproof plasters
- Sterile dressings

First aid kit

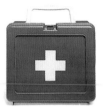

Keep first aid kits in your car and in your home. You can buy kits ready made up. You may want to add extra dressings and bandages or specialist plasters – blister plasters, for example. Make sure the first aid box is readily accessible and easy to identify, and check the contents regularly. Do not keep medicines in the same box; they should be locked in a medicine cabinet. A well-stocked kit might contain the articles shown here. *See p.108 for alternative household items.*

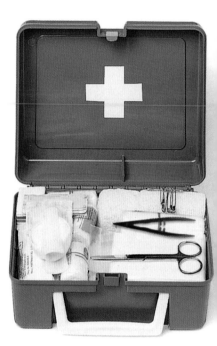

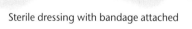

Blunt-ended scissors

Plastic tweezers

Dressings

Plasters (adhesive dressings) are used for minor wounds. Keep several different sizes and shapes, including a selection of larger sterile dressings for more serious wounds.

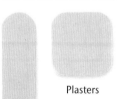

Plasters

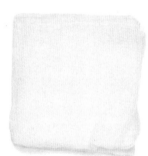

Gauze swabs

Sterile non-adhesive pad

Sterile dressing with bandage attached

Bandages

Keep a variety of bandages to secure dressings and support injured joints. Conforming bandages shape themselves to the contours of the body and so are easy to use. Triangular bandages can be used as slings and for broad- and narrow-fold bandages.

Tape for securing dressings

Small conforming bandage

Large conforming bandage

Bandage clip

Safety pins for securing bandages

Tube-gauze finger bandage and applicator

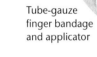

Bandage slides over applicator

Folded triangular bandage

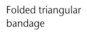

Additional useful equipment

- If you have a note pad and pen or pencil you can write down important information about a child's condition to give to the emergency services.
- Keep a torch beside your home first aid kit (for use in the event of a power failure), and in your car; check and replace the batteries regularly.
- Plastic face shields or face masks can protect you and a child from cross infection when you are giving rescue breaths.
- Keep a plastic or foil emergency survival blanket or bag in your car.
- Always carry a warning triangle in your car and place it in the road behind the car in the event of a breakdown or crash.

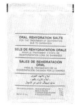

ORAL REHYDRATION SALTS

Sachets of rehydration salts are added to water. Use them to treat dehydration resulting from heat exhaustion or vomiting.

INSTANT ICE PACKS

Keep a pack of these in the car - they are especially useful when you do not have access to a freezer.

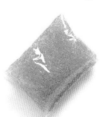

Digital thermometer

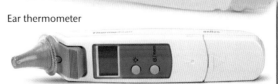

Ear thermometer

THERMOMETER

Choose one with an easy-to-read screen. Check the battery regularly.

Dressings

Covering a wound helps the blood-clotting process and prevents infection. Dressings should not be fluffy and must be large enough to cover the wound and area around it. Wash your hands before applying dressings and wear disposable gloves if possible. If blood soaks through a dressing, place another on top. Make sure bandages are not too tight (*see opposite*).

Plaster

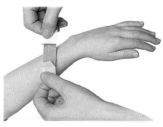

Remove wrapping and, holding the pad over the wound, peel back the protective strips. Press the ends and edges down.

Sterile pad

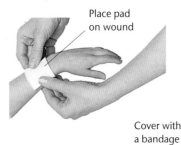

Place pad on wound

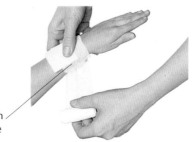

Cover with a bandage

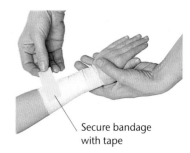

Secure bandage with tape

1 Place the dressing pad shiny-side down directly over the child's wound.

2 Secure the pad with a bandage, working from below the injury up the limb.

3 Secure the end of the bandage with strips of hypoallergenic tape.

Sterile dressing with bandage

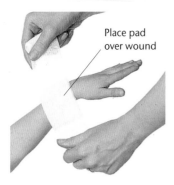

Place pad over wound

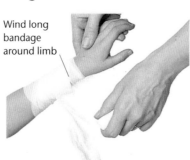

Wind long bandage around limb

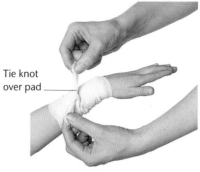

Tie knot over pad

1 Hold the bandage either side of the dressing pad, and place the pad over the wound.

2 Leaving the short end hanging, wind the other end around the limb to cover dressing.

3 Tie the two ends of the bandage in a knot directly over the pad.

Bandaging

Use bandages to secure dressings, to help control bleeding, and to support injuries. Roller bandages can be used for any part of the body; conforming bandages are especially useful for bandaging joints or head wounds as they mould themselves to the shape of the body.

Check circulation

Do not apply a bandage too tightly – it will impair the circulation. To check, press on your child's nail or a patch of skin beyond the bandage, then release pressure. The colour should return rapidly. If it does not, loosen the bandages.

Roller bandage

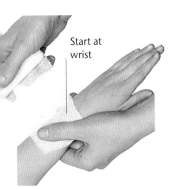

Start at wrist

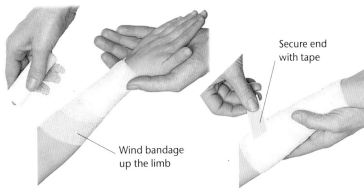

Wind bandage up the limb

Secure end with tape

1 Place the end of the bandage on the arm below the injury and hold the bandage roll in your other hand.

2 Still supporting the injured limb, wind the bandage around the arm, working up the limb. Stop above the injury.

3 Make two straight turns to finish. Secure the end with tape. Check circulation in your child's fingers (*see above*).

Hand bandage

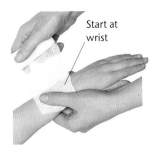

Start at wrist

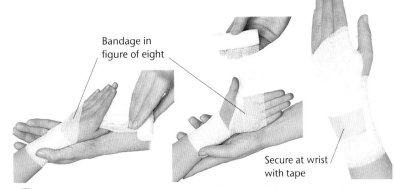

Bandage in figure of eight

Secure at wrist with tape

1 Supporting the injured hand, hold the end of the bandage on the wrist and make two straight turns around the wrist.

2 Take the bandage across the back of the hand to the base of the little finger. Then take it around the palm, up between the thumb and forefinger, and across the back of the hand to the wrist. Repeat the figure of eight to cover the hand. Check circulation.

Triangular bandages

These are sold singly in sterile packs or can be made from a 1m (39in) square of strong fabric folded diagonally in half. Triangular bandages are used for slings or to make broad-fold and narrow-fold bandages (*see p.65*) to immobilise an injured leg or for extra support around a sling. Arm slings support injured arms or wrists, or take weight off an injured shoulder. Elevation slings are used to support hand injuries to minimise bleeding, pain, or swelling.

Arm sling

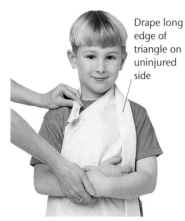

Drape long edge of triangle on uninjured side

1 Place the bandage between your child's arm and chest, easing one end up around the back of his neck on the injured side.

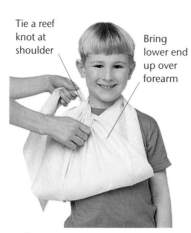

Tie a reef knot at shoulder

Bring lower end up over forearm

2 Take the lower end of the bandage up over your child's forearm to the end at the shoulder and tie a knot just below the shoulder.

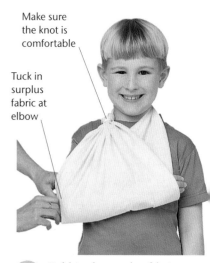

Make sure the knot is comfortable

Tuck in surplus fabric at elbow

3 Fold in the surplus fabric at the corner near the elbow and pin it to the bandage.

Improvised slings

If your child injures her shoulder, arm, or hand, you can make an improvised sling to support the injury until she receives medical treatment.

● Undo a coat or shirt button and tuck the hand of the injured arm inside the fastening – don't use this method if the child's forearm or wrist is injured.

● Pin your child's sleeve up on the opposite side of his chest.

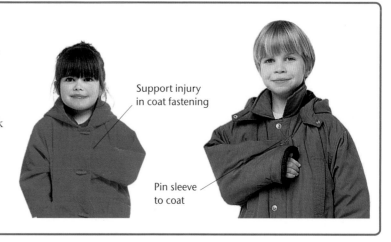

Support injury in coat fastening

Pin sleeve to coat

Elevation sling

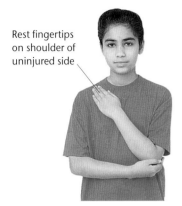

Rest fingertips on shoulder of uninjured side

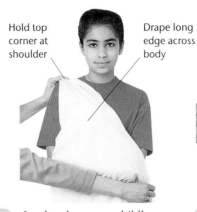

Hold top corner at shoulder

Drape long edge across body

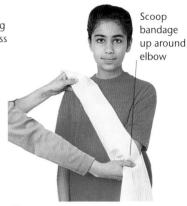

Scoop bandage up around elbow

1 Bring the arm on the injured side across your child's chest. Ask her to support her elbow.

2 Lay bandage over child's arm, with longest edge on the uninjured side. Hold the top corner.

3 Support the child's arm and fold long edge of bandage in under injured arm.

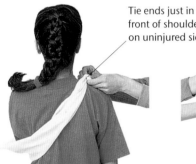

Tie ends just in front of shoulder on uninjured side

4 Bring the lower end up around her back, holding the elbow securely in the fabric. Tie a knot just below the shoulder and tuck the ends in.

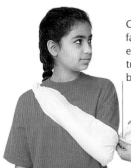

Gather slack fabric at elbow and tuck in behind

OR

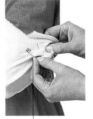

Pin slack fabric to front of sling

5 Secure the sling by twisting the excess fabric and tucking it in at the elbow or fold and pin in place.

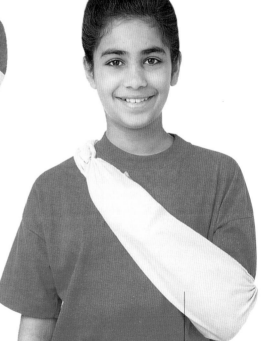

Finished sling raises, immobilises, and supports the injury

Useful household items

You should keep a well-stocked first aid kit (*see p.102*) both at home and in the car. However, there are many everyday items around the home that are invaluable for first aid emergencies.

- Plastic credit cards can be used to scrape off an insect sting (*see p.80*).
- A tea towel can be used as a pad to control bleeding or as an improvised dressing or to secure a dressing.
- Use vinegar to treat a jellyfish sting (*see p.82*) – it neutralizes the effect of the sting and prevents it from spreading.
- Beer or milk can be used to cool a burn if there is no cold water available (*see p.52*).
- Milk stops a knocked-out adult tooth drying out while you get the child to a dentist (*see p.47*).
- Use a telephone directory, thick book, or wooden box as insulation when dealing with electrical injury (*see p.12*).

Making a cold pack

- Packs of frozen vegetables or fruit such as peas, raspberries, or currants make ideal ice packs as the bags mould to the shape of the body and stay cool for a long time. Wrap it in cloth before putting on your child for up to 20 minutes.

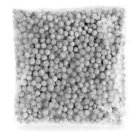

- Fill a sandwich or freezer bag two-thirds full of ice, then seal the bag; and wrap it in cloth before putting on your child for 20 minutes.

Frozen peas in a plastic bag

- Soak a flannel in cold water, wring out the excess water, then place it over the injury for 20 minutes.

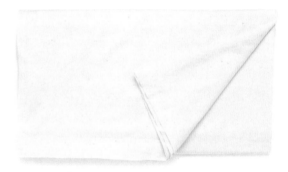

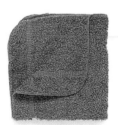

FLANNEL
Use a flannel soaked in cold water to make a cold pack as well as to clean up a child after an incident.

SHEETS AND PILLOW CASES
A clean cotton sheet or pillowcase makes an excellent loose protective covering for burns.

PLASTIC BAGS
A clean plastic bag can be put over a burned foot or hand and lightly secured with bandages or tape. Always cool the burn first.

CLING FILM
Cover cooled burns with plastic kitchen film to protect from infection.

Safety at home

Most incidents occur at home and over half involve children under the age of five. Many incidents are preventable if you:

- Plan the layout and position of objects and furniture at home with child safety in mind.
- Make sure that all windows are closed or inaccessible (don't leave chairs beside them).
- Never confuse containers by putting a dangerous substance, such as bleach, in a bottle that used to contain a harmless drink.
- Install smoke alarms, carbon monoxide alarms, fire guards, and safety gates in your home.
- Never pretend that medicines and pills are special sweets to encourage a child to take medication. Keep all medicines locked away.
- Check for hazards when visiting friends and ask if you can move sharp or breakable objects.
- Teach your child basic safety rules.

Fire

If fire breaks out at home, it could be a matter of minutes before smoke overcomes you.

- Fit smoke alarms throughout your home. If your home is on one level, fit a detector between the sitting room and the bedrooms. If your house has two or more levels, fit detectors at the foot of the stairs and on every floor outside the bedrooms; ideally they should be linked. If you live in an apartment block there should be detectors in all communal areas too.
- Test smoke alarms regularly; replace batteries if they have them.
- Have an escape plan (*see p.11*). Make sure the whole family knows what to do if there is a fire, especially at night. Practise the fire drill with your children: shout "fire"; tell everyone to drop to the floor if there is smoke and crawl to the nearest exit from the rooms; shut each door behind you; arrange a meeting point outside where everyone should wait together. Don't go back for pets or treasured possessions.

Electricity

Protect your child from electric shock (*see p.12*) or fire caused by electric faults.

- Cover sockets – put heavy furniture in front of them.
- Use bar-type fused adaptors with surge protectors on extension leads instead of block-type socket adaptors.
- Wire plugs correctly – follow instructions and check that you have the right fuse.
- Replace worn or damaged flexes.
- Tidy up trailing wires to prevent tripping hazards.
- Unplug electrical appliances at night, particularly the televisions and computers.
- Fit an RCD (residual current device) to power tools.

Gas

Fit carbon monoxide alarms and have all boilers and gas appliances serviced regularly. Find out where your main gas tap is in case there is a leak. If you smell gas call 0800 111 999:

- Don't turn lights or electric switches on or off – there may be a spark, which can cause an explosion.
- Don't light matches or cigarettes.
- Turn off the mains gas tap and open the windows.

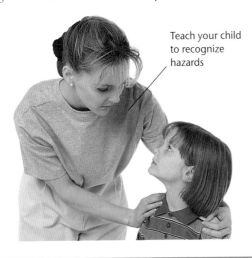

Teach your child to recognize hazards

Hall and stairs

The staircase is not a safe place for your child to play (*see below*).

- Make sure that toys are not left on the stairs for you to trip over.
- Put a light in your hall or on the landing so that your child can see if he gets up at night.

If you don't want the area too light, use a low-watt bulb. Never cover a lamp with a cloth as the cloth can easily catch fire.

- Don't let your child play on the landings or stairs of a communal area in flats as the banisters may have large gaps between them.

Front and back doors

- Never leave your front door open.
- Don't let your child answer the door to callers.
- Put the door catch out of reach of small children. If your toddler can reach the catch, fix an additional bolt higher up the door and keep the door bolted.
- If the door has a deadlock that needs a key to open, make sure that the key is accessible to adults and older children so that they can escape if there's a fire.
- Fit toughened or laminated glass in doors that have glass within 80cm (2ft 8in) of the floor. If this is not possible stick plastic safety film over it as it can prevent the glass splintering if it is broken. Put stickers over the glass to make it more noticeable, especially for young children.

Floors

Tiled, polished, laminated, or hessian-covered floors can be very slippery for toddlers and running children.

- Put non-slip webbing under rugs.
- Keep hall floors free of toys and clutter.
- Check fitted carpets regularly for holes or loose carpet that might trip you or your toddler.

Stairs

A child is not coordinated enough to be able to walk downstairs safely until he is at least three years old.

- Fit safety gates at the foot of the stairs and across the upper landing or across your child's bedroom doorway (safety gates at the top of the stairs can be a trip hazard). Safety gates should comply with British Standard EN 1930:2011 so the bars must be no more than 5.5cm (2⅛in) apart and avoid stair gates that open leaving a bar across the base as they are a trip hazard. Always open the gate; never climb over it as your child will copy you.
- Check your banisters regularly: the handrail and posts should be secured. Posts should not be too far apart – anything wider than 6.5cm (2½in) apart should be boarded up. Don't let your child climb banisters. If the stairs or landing has horizontal rails (so-called ranch-type banisters), they should be boarded up because it is very easy for a child to climb them.
- Replace loose or worn carpet or steps. They are trip hazards.

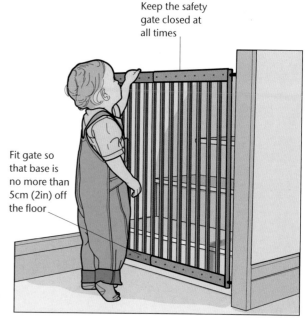

Keep the safety gate closed at all times

Fit gate so that base is no more than 5cm (2in) off the floor

Sitting room

While your children are very young, try to arrange the room so that both children and your valuables are kept out of harm's way.

- If you have a balcony, ensure that it is too high for your child to climb. Block up gaps in the railings with hardboard.
- Fit safety glass in patio doors if the glass is within 80cm (2ft 8in) of the floor.

Carpets and curtains

- Check that there are no areas of carpet or rug that have holes or turned-up edges; either you or your child could trip up.
- Wind up and tuck away all curtain ties and pull cords for blinds. Children can be strangled if they get caught in dangling cords.

Fireplaces and heaters

- Don't leave matches or cigarette lighters where your child can reach them.
- Cover all fires with a fireguard. Fix the guard to the wall to prevent your child pulling it over.
- Use a spark-guard as well as a fireguard for open solid fuel fires as an additional precaution.
- Never use the fireguard as a shelf or clothes airer.

Electrical equipment

- Fix wiring to the skirting boards.
- Run long flexes behind furniture so that your child can't trip or pull on them.
- Replace items with worn flexes.
- If your TV is on a stand ensure that it is secure and cannot be pulled over. Ideally fix the TV to the wall.

Surfaces and furniture

- Place house plants out of reach of young children. Dispose of any poisonous plants. Some can scratch or produce allergic reactions if touched.
- Do not place breakable or heavy objects on low tables. Set them well back from the edges of surfaces such as window sills or mantelpieces.
- Glass-topped tables should comply with BS EN 12521:2015. Put protectors on sharp table corners.
- Don't leave hot drinks, alcohol, glasses, cigarettes, matches, or lighters on low surfaces, such as coffee tables, where your child can reach them.
- Keep alcohol in a locked cupboard.
- Never leave a cigarette burning in an ashtray on the arm of a sofa or armchair.
- Make sure all sofas and armchairs have a fire safety label; old foam furniture is lethal in a fire.

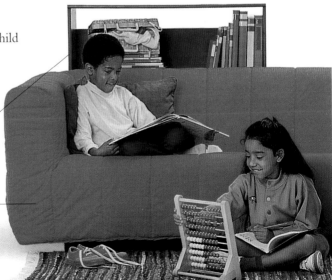

Ensure bookcases are secured to the wall

Sofas and armchairs must have fire-resistant fillings and coverings

Kitchen

This is the busiest part of your house, where you spend a lot of time with your children.

- Never hold baby or child in your arms when you are cooking or carrying a hot drink.

Doors

- Fit safety glass to any glass panels. Cover glass panels within 80cm (2ft 8in) of the floor with safety film, to stop glass shattering or splintering if broken.
- Put some colourful stickers on the glass door panels to alert your child.

Floors

- Create a safe play area away from where you work. Don't let your child play between you and the work surface or anywhere you could trip over him.
- Avoid bumps and falls by wiping up spills immediately.
- Remove pet food bowls after use and keep that part of the floor scrupulously clean.
- Keep a box for tidying away toys and clutter.

Wastebins

- Discourage toddlers from rummaging in the wastebin.
- Put sharp-edged cans and lids or broken glass straight into the dustbin outside.
- Keep the wastebin in a cupboard with a child-resistant safety catch.

> **! IMPORTANT**
>
> - Keep a fire blanket in the kitchen for smothering flare-ups. If you want to buy a fire extinguisher, consult your local fire brigade to find out which is the most appropriate type. Check fire extinguisher regularly. For more on fires, *see p.11 and p.109.*

Babies in the kitchen

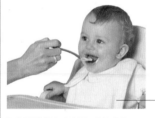

Stay with your child when he is eating in case he chokes

BOTTLES AND FOOD

- Sterilise all your baby's feeding equipment, or put it in a dishwasher.
- Don't leave a prepared feed standing at room temperature, and don't keep the remains of the last feed. Warmed and reheated feeds are breeding grounds for bacteria.
- Make fresh bottles for each feed;

don't prepare them in advance and re-heat them. Check the temperature before you feed your baby.

HIGHCHAIRS

- Always use the safety harness.
- Never leave the highchair where your baby can reach out and pull objects down from a surface.
- Never leave your child unattended in a highchair.

PLAY

- Put your baby in a playpen away from the cooking area, or put a gate across the doorway.
- Keep him out of range of any spills from the cooker.

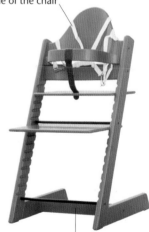

Attach a safety harness to the clips on either side of the chair

Choose a stable highchair with widely spaced legs

Tables and work surfaces

- Always be aware of your child's reach and keep all heavy, breakable, or sharp objects well back from the edges of work surfaces.
- Keep stools or chairs away from tables and kitchen work surfaces to prevent a young child from climbing up on them.
- Tuck flexes of kettles, toasters, blenders, and irons out of reach. Choose a curly flex for your kettle if possible. It is not only boiling, steaming kettles that pose a hazard: the water in a kettle is still hot enough to scald 15 minutes after boiling.
- Leave all electrical appliances unplugged when they are not in use.
- Avoid using a tablecloth. It is tempting for a crawling baby or toddler to use it to pull himself up, bringing anything on the table down upon his head. Use table mats instead, or secure the cloth with clips.
- Do not put your baby on a table or work surface when he is in a car seat or bouncing cradle – he could easily bounce himself off.

Cupboards and drawers

- Put safety catches on cupboards and drawers, particularly those containing: matches, lighters, knives, scissors, and cutlery; heavy pots, pans, or china; dried food, such as lentils or pasta, which may be a choking hazard; bottles containing alcohol; medicines; cleaning materials, such as washing powder, or dishwasher detergent, even if fitted with "child-resistant" lids.

Fridges

Food poisoning can be caused by poor food storage. Take precautions to minimise risks:

- Keep cooked meat and poultry on a separate shelf from uncooked meat. Cover uncooked meat with kitchen film.
- Don't store food in open tins; tip leftovers into a clean container, cover, and put in the fridge.
- Check food regularly to see that nothing is kept beyond the "use-by" date.

Cookers

Your child is obviously at risk of burns and scalds from hot fat or boiling water when you are preparing food.

- You can buy safety guards, but remember that a child can still poke fingers through some types and be burned by hot hobs or gas rings.
- Always keep your child away from oven doors; they can get very hot while the oven is in use and will stay hot for some time afterwards. A crawling baby or toddler is particularly at risk. Try to teach your child what "hot" means so that he understands a warning.
- Keep ingintion devices, matches, and lighters well out of reach in a cupboard fitted with a safety catch.

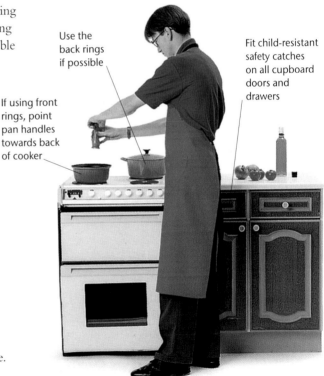

Use the back rings if possible

If using front rings, point pan handles towards back of cooker

Fit child-resistant safety catches on all cupboard doors and drawers

Washing and drying machines

- Keep small hands away from the glass door; it may get hot while the machine is on.
- Ensure the door is closed when the machines are not in use. Your toddler may try to climb inside or even fill it with toys.

Bedrooms

The cupboards and drawers in bedrooms are always exciting places for toddlers and young children. Make sure any potentially hazardous items are out of reach, as you may not always know when your child will decide to go exploring on his own.

Baby's cots

- Make sure the cot is deep enough to prevent your baby from climbing out – at least 50cm (1ft 8in) from the top of the mattress to the top of the cot.

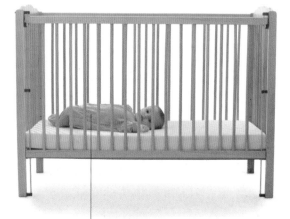

Put your baby down to sleep with her feet at the base of the cot

- Bar spaces must be between 2.5 and 6cm (1–2½in) wide to prevent your baby's head from being trapped.
- The mattress must fit the cot with a gap of less than 3cm (1½in) around the side or the baby's head could become trapped between the cot side and the mattress.
- Don't use a pillow for a baby under one year: it could suffocate him. If you need to raise his head, put a pillow under the mattress or raise one end of the cot.
- Use a sheet and cellular blankets rather than a duvet until your baby is one year old. Your baby could overheat or suffocate under a duvet.
- Don't put the cot near a radiator or in a very sunny part of the room. Don't use a cot bumper.
- Put your baby to sleep on his back with his feet at the foot of the cot to lessen the risk of cot death; babies under 6 months should sleep in their parent's room.
- Remove toys from the cot as soon as your baby can sit up because he could use them to climb out.
- Once your child starts trying to climb out of the cot, transfer him to a bed.

Changing areas

- Keep all changing equipment in one place so that you never have to leave your baby alone on the changing mat. He will be safest on the floor, but if you have a changing table, remember that he might roll off if left even for a moment.
- Store nappy sacs well out of the reach of babies as these present a suffocation risk.
- Do not have shelves above the changing area in case something falls off onto your child.
- Keep dangling mobiles out of his reach.
- Use a towel rather than talcum powder to dry your baby's skin as the fine particles can be harmful if your baby breathes in lots of them at once.

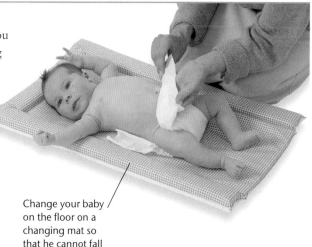

Change your baby on the floor on a changing mat so that he cannot fall

Children's bedrooms

This is a room where where children are likely to be unsupervised so they have to be as safe as possible.

- All blinds and curtain mechanisms should comply with EN13120:2009+ A1:2014. Ideally choose blinds without a loop mechanism, but if there is one fitted it must have a safety release that breaks under pressure. Stow curtain ties well out of reach of children.
- Don't use a bed guard when your toddler first moves to a bed; if you think he may fall out, put cushions on the floor beside the bed.
- A top bunk bed is not recommended for children under the age of six.
- Top bunk beds must have safety rails on both sides and any gaps in the railings or between the top of the mattress and the bottom of the safety rail should be no more than 6–7.5cm (2½–3in).
- Never let young children play on the top bunk.
- Remove toys from the floor by the bed at night.
- Ensure there are no wires near a child's bed.

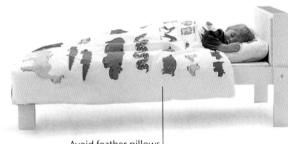

Avoid feather pillows and duvets as they can provoke allergies

WINDOWS

Make sure your child can't climb out of the window. He is in danger even if his room is on the ground floor.

- Fix a safety catch, but make sure the window can be opened easily in the event of a fire.
- Don't place a piece of furniture below a window because it may encourage your child to climb up.

TOYS *(see also p.117)*

- Keep toys that are unsuitable for very young children separate from others. This way you can easily put them out of reach if your child is sharing a room with a younger child, or if you have young visitors.

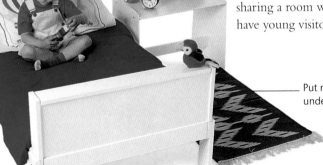

Put non-slip webbing under rugs

Your bedroom

The Lullaby Trust advises that babies under 6 months should sleep in a cot in their parent's room – although not in a parent's bed.

- Perfume, hairspray, and makeup can be harmful if sprayed or rubbed in the eyes, or swallowed, so keep them out of reach or in a drawer with a safety catch.
- Medicines and pills should never be left beside your bed, or on a dressing table. Put them out of sight and out of a child's reach, preferably in a locked cupboard.
- Scissors and sewing equipment should be kept in a drawer or cupboard with a safety catch.
- Never leave a china cup or a glass on the floor by your bed, especially at night. If your child happened to be in your bed he could roll out onto the cup or the glass.

Bathroom

Your child may be at risk from falls, drowning, scalding, or poisoning in the bathroom. Keep the door shut at all times to discourage him from going in. If you install a bolt on the door, fix it towards the top of the door to prevent a young child locking himself in.

Baths

- Check the temperature of the water before your child gets into the bath. Put your elbow in the water; if it is too hot for your elbow it is too hot for your child. A child can be badly scalded by hot bathwater.
- Fit thermostatic mixing valves to the hot taps to limit the temperature of water from the tap.
- Place non-slip mats in the bath and on the floor beside the bath.
- Keep babies and toddlers away from the bath taps.
- Never leave a young child or baby alone in the bath (or in the care of another child). A baby can drown in just 2.5cm (1in) of water. If you need to answer the door or telephone, take your baby with you.

Showers

- Keep a constant check on the temperature of the water.
- Use non-slip mats in the shower and on the bathroom floor.
- Fix safety film on a glass shower door so that glass is held in place in case of an incident.

Cupboards and cabinets

- Store bathroom chemicals and other potential poisons, such as toilet cleaners and bleach, out of reach in a cupboard with a safety catch.
- Keep other hazards, such as make-up, aftershave, razors, nail scissors, and any medicines or glass containers, out of reach in a locked medicine cabinet.

Toilets

- Use a special child toilet seat adaptor and step for toddlers so that they can keep their balance more easily and so feel more secure.
- Keep the toilet seat closed when not in use.
- Don't use block toilet cleaners that a young child could pull out and chew.
- Never use toilet cleaners as well as bleach as this will produce toxic fumes.
- If your toddler uses a potty, keep it clean, but never leave bleach or cleaning agents inside it.

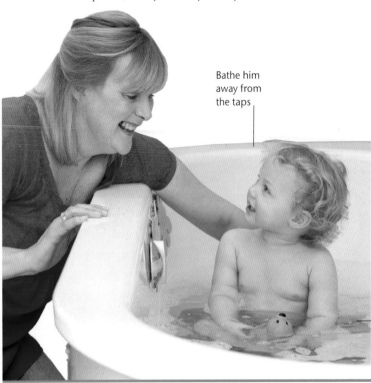

Bathe him away from the taps

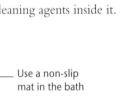

Use a non-slip mat in the bath

Toys and playthings

If you have children of different ages in your home, keep their toys in separate boxes. In particular, keep toys with small parts away from younger children.

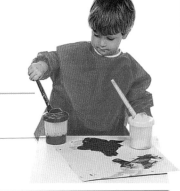

Choosing toys

- Buy toys that are appropriate for the age of your child, and buy from a reputable source.
- Don't give your child anything to play with that has sharp edges, or is made of thin, rigid plastic.
- Give him non-toxic paints or crayons.
- Don't buy your child old second-hand toys: they may be broken or covered in paint containing lead.

Give your child non-toxic paints to play with

- Avoid novelty toys that are not designed to be played with by young children: look out for warnings on the packaging.

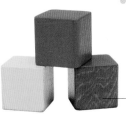

Check sets of building blocks for small pieces that could be a choking hazard for a younger child

Caring for toys

- Check toys regularly and always throw away any broken ones.
- Don't mix old and new batteries. Change them all at the same time, otherwise the strong batteries will make the weak ones very hot.
- Keep toys in a toy box. Toys can bring about accidents and injuries if left on the floor.

Babies and toddlers

- Remove ribbons from a baby's soft toys.
- Check that the eyes, noses, ears, or bells on soft toys and dolls are well secured.
- Attach cot toys with a very short string and remove them as soon as your baby can sit up.
- Remove activity centres or bulky toys from a cot as soon as your child can stand because they provide a foothold for climbing out of the cot.
- Don't let babies chew on furry toys: the fur is a choking hazard.
- Never let a young child play with a toy that is not recommended for his age-group: it may contain small pieces on which he could choke.
- Don't leave a baby or toddler to play in a room on his own.
- Baby walkers serve no useful purpose. If you do use one, make sure it complies with BS EN 1273: 2005. Older walkers can tip over, and can be dangerous for your baby.

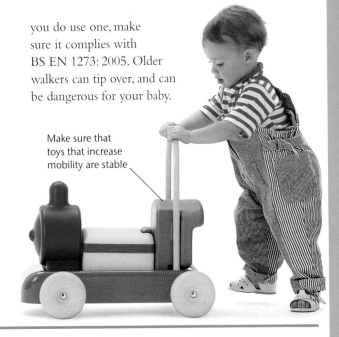

Make sure that toys that increase mobility are stable

Garden

Your garden can be a safe and interesting place for your children to play. Children will find their own corners to play in but you must clear away rubbish and remove obvious hazards:

- Lock gates that lead out of the garden and make sure fences are secure.
- Check garden furniture or play equipment regularly to make sure that it is safe. Site it over grass not paving stones.
- Keep pets away from children's play areas.
- Make sure paving is even and remove moss so neither you or your child trip or slip.

Plants

Many plants are poisonous if eaten and digested in large quantities. Small pieces, or one or two berries, are not fatal but may cause some discomfort and stomach upset.

- Tell your child about the dangers of eating berries, and keep babies and toddlers away from them.
- Remove plants that you know to be poisonous, such as deadly nightshade, laburnum, and toadstools.
- Cut back any prickly plants, such as roses, brambles, and holly. They can give nasty scratches, especially to your or your child's eyes.

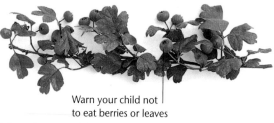

Warn your child not to eat berries or leaves

Sheds and bins

Sheds are inevitably used for storing chemical and tools. and so are a potential hazard.

- Tell your child that the shed is out of bounds, keep it locked at all times, and hide the key.
- Put chemicals, such as weedkiller or slug pellets, out of reach in containers with child-resistant tops.
- Keep wheelie bins hinge side outwards so a child can't open them and climb in.

Water in the garden

Babies and toddlers are especially at risk if they slip and fall, even in shallow water. Maintain fencing to prevent children entering a neighbour's garden where a pond may be a hazard.

- Never leave children unattended when they are playing in, or near, water.
- Keep ponds covered and fenced off, and cover water butts and empty dustbins that collect rainwater.
- Always empty out a paddling pool when your children have finished playing in it and turn it upside-down in case it rains.

Gardening

- Don't put down chemicals when children will be playing in the garden.
- Don't mow the lawn while children are close by because stone chips may become dislodged and fly up into their eyes.
- Put away all garden tools when you have finished using them.

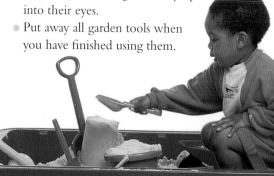

Check that he is playing in a clean, safe area with safe toys

Garage and car safety

Always leave your garage locked; likewise keep the car locked, even if it is on a driveway off the road or in a garage. Keep the car keys where the children cannot reach them. Don't give the keys to your baby to play with as they are not clean and he could drop them.

Garages and drives

- Keep the garage locked and discourage your child from going in there.
- Keep equipment, chemicals, or tools out of your child's reach and locked away if possible.
- Make sure you know where your child is when you are driving into, or out of, the garage or a drive.
- If you keep a deep freeze in the garage, it should be locked at all times.

Cars

- Never leave a young child unattended in a car, even if you can see the car.
- Don't let your child play with the car windows, whether manual or electric. Windows can trap a child's head or fingers.
- Remove the cigarette lighter from the car altogether.
- Watch out for your child's fingers when you shut the car doors.
- Use child locks on rear doors until your child is at least six years old.
- Teach your child to get out of the car on the pavement side.
- If your child is helping you wash the car, make sure you have removed the car keys from the ignition first.

Car seats

Always put your child into a special safety seat when you strap him into the car. The law requires that all children up to 135cm (about 4ft 5in) travelling in cars use a child restraint – in some countries this limit is 150cm (4ft 11in). Never carry a baby or child on your lap even in your seatbelt – it is not only dangerous (your baby could be thrown out of the car or crushed by your body weight in a crash) but it is also illegal.

There are various types of car seat – the correct one will depend on the age or your baby or child and your car. Ideally when you buy a seat, go to a retailer who will allow you to try it in your car before you buy it, and show you how to use it properly. Fit the seat exactly as the instructions describe. Most cars now have special Isofix seat fixings for child car seats and connectors on the seats clip onto these fixings. Check that your chosen Isofix seat is approved for use in your particular vehicle; Isofix seats will not fit in every car with Isofix points. Then choose the correct seat for the weight and development of your child:

- Babies up to 13kg (29lb) – about 12–15 months – should travel in a rear-facing car seat. The safest place for your baby to travel is on the rear seat of your car. Do not place your baby in a rear-facing car seat on the front passenger seat if there is an airbag fitted that cannot be disabled – the impact of an airbag inflating could cause serious injury.
- Older babies and toddlers, up to 18kg (40lb), need a car seat in the back of the car. Some seats have an integral harness for the child, which fits over his shoulders, across his hips, and between his legs. The seats are held in place by the Isofix fixings, an adult seat belt, or straps that you fix into the car.
- Children who weigh more than more than 22kg (48lbs) can travel in a booster seat. Without them, adult seat belts are neither comfortable nor safe: the shoulder part cuts across the child's neck, and the lap strap lies across his stomach, which could cause internal injury in a crash. A lap strap on its own is not sufficient as it does not restrain the child's upper body.

Finally, use a seat on every journey in a car, no matter how short - even in taxis.

Out and about

After the home, most childhood incidents occur in the street or in play areas. Teach your child the rules of the road from an early age, reminding him to stay alert for traffic and to cross in a safe place. It takes a long time for children to develop a true road sense.

What a child understands
- Three-year-olds can learn that the pavement is safe and the road is dangerous.
- Five-year-olds can learn how to cross the road, but they are still not able to put this knowledge into practice on their own.
- Eight-year-olds can cross quiet streets on their own, but they are not yet able to judge the speed and distance of traffic.
- Twelve-year-olds can judge the speed of an oncoming car, but are still easily distracted by friends.

Street and road safety
Whenever you are out with your child, show him how to be aware of his own safety.
- When out shopping or walking near a road, use reins or a wrist strap for a toddler, to stop him running off without you.
- Encourage a young child to hold your hand when you are near the road or waiting to cross a road.

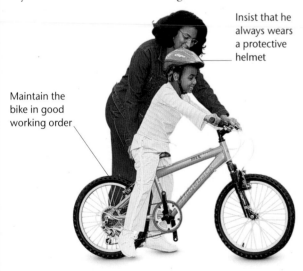

Insist that he always wears a protective helmet

Maintain the bike in good working order

Learning how to cross the road
Teach your child the rules of the road:
- Find a safe place to cross, then stop.
- Stand on the pavement, near the kerb.
- Look all around for traffic, and listen.
- If traffic is coming, let it pass.
- When there is no traffic near, walk straight across the road.
- Look and listen for traffic while you cross.

- Teach your child by example and always find a safe place to cross a road. This may be a zebra crossing, a pelican crossing with lights, an underpass, or a footbridge. If there is no designated crossing point, aim for a large gap between parked cars, where you and your child can see a long way in both directions.
- At a zebra crossing teach your child to stop and wait until all the traffic has stopped and to stop at the island halfway across, if there is one.
- When using a pedestrian crossing with traffic lights, encourage your child to press the button and always wait until the traffic has stopped before crossing.

Bikes
- All children should wear a helmet when riding a bike.
- Children under 10 years old should not cycle on roads in traffic without an adult and all children should have cycle training before going on the road.
- Make sure your child can be seen when he's riding his bike – with bright fluorescent colours by day and reflectors on his clothes and bike by night.

Where to play

What may seem common sense to you is not obvious to children.

- Show your child where it is safe to play – the playground, or local recreation ground, for example – and supervise him if necessary.
- Teach your child the dangers of playing in open areas, such as roads, building sites, and quarries.
- Tell your child not to play in the street, or on a pavement near the kerb – even if your street is quiet.
- Tell him that he must never chase a ball, a pet, or another child into the road.

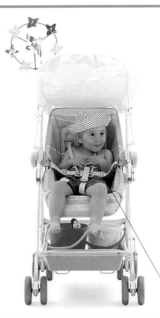

Harness your baby into his buggy

Prams and buggies

- Never push a pram or buggy out into the traffic to see if the road is clear to cross. Pull the buggy to one side and check whether the road is safe. Remember that a child's buggy sticks out in front of you by at least 1m (3ft).
- When you park a pram or buggy, put on the brakes and point it away from traffic.
- Never tie your dog to the pram.
- Never leave a baby unattended.
- Keep your child away from the buggy when you are assembling or folding it to keep little fingers from being trapped.

In the playground

All playgrounds should comply with safety standards; report any faulty equipment in community playgrounds to your local authority.

- The play area must be safely fenced off and away from roads.
- There should be a soft, even surface, such as bark chippings or rubber tiles, around equipment.
- Slides should be no higher than 2.4m (8ft) and preferably constructed on an earth mound to break any falls.
- Roundabouts should be low, with a smooth surface, designed so that young children can't get their feet stuck underneath.
- Climbing frames should be no higher than 2.4m (8ft), completely stable, and built over sand or a very soft surface to break falls.
- Swings should set away from main play equipment.
- There should be a clearly defined play area for toddlers and young children, set away from the more boisterous activities of older children.
- There should be someone to contact if any of the equipment is faulty.
- Dogs must not be allowed inside playgrounds.

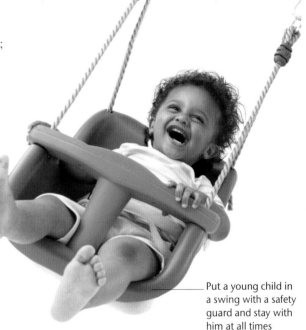

Put a young child in a swing with a safety guard and stay with him at all times

 IMPORTANT

- **Remind** your child of the dangers of talking to strangers. Have a code word that a friend can use if colllecting your child. Tell your child not to go with anybody unless they use the code.

Travelling with babies and children

Away from your home all the same rules of safety apply. However, you should be aware that the place you are staying in would not necessarily have been planned with young children in mind.

- If there is a swimming pool, never leave your child unattended in or near the water and, if there is a fence around it, keep the gate shut.
- Take baby milk and/or food with you as your child may not like what is available locally.

Travelling abroad

- Make sure your child's immunisations are up to date. Some countries recommend additional vaccination, or anti-malaria medication; ask when booking a trip.
- Don't forget to take the necessary paperwork; babies and children need their own passports for most countries. It is a good idea to keep a photocopy of each passport (yours as well) in a separate bag.
- If you are hiring a car, always ask for child safety seats, or take your child's car seat with you.
- Make sure hire cars are fitted with sufficient safety belts and check that they are in good condition (not frayed) and working properly.
- Take insect repellent suitable for babies and young children, as they are particularly susceptible to insect bites. Apply the repellant in the early evening and again at bedtime when the insects are most active.
- Wash vegetables, salads, and fruit in cooled, boiled water or bottled water if there is any doubt about the local water.
- Boil water used to make up baby foods or milk.

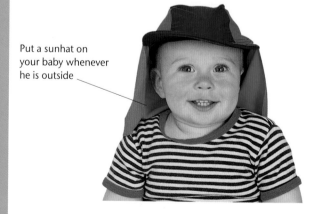

Put a sunhat on your baby whenever he is outside

Air travel

- If booking tickets for children under the age of two, ask for seats where you can use a child safety seat or ask the airline if they can provide a sky cot.
- Give your baby a breastfeed, bottlefeed, or a dummy to suck as the plane ascends and descends because the change in pressure can cause earache in babies and children. Give an older child a sweet to suck, but make sure he does not choke on it.
- Take any food or milk that a baby needs on the journey. Airlines don't generally carry baby food, though they may be able to heat yours for you.
- Give your baby or child plenty to drink during the flight to prevent dehydration.

Sun protection

- Use sun block that protects your child from ultra violet A rays (UVA) and ultra violet B rays (UVB). The sun protector factor (SPF) numbers relate to UVA – chose SPF 30 – and a star-rating system indicates UVB protection. Re-apply regularly, especially after he has been in water. Use a cream that you know your child is not allergic to.
- Keep your baby or child's arms and legs covered as much as possible. Dress him in clothes made of closely woven fabric made of natural fibres.
- Make sure your child is protected by the shade in the middle of the day (about 10am until 4pm).
- Put a wide-brimmed hat on your child's head that covers his neck and face and use a parasol on a buggy.
- Give your child plenty to drink to prevent dehydration. If you are breastfeeding offer your baby more feeds; give a bottlefed baby plain water.

Index

A

abdominal wound 51
adhesive dressings 102
adrenaline, Epipen 91
AED, paediatric, 23
air travel 122
   pressure-change earache 100
airway
   anaphylactic shock 91
   blocked 17
   resuscitation 17
   unresponsive baby 19
   unresponsive child 22
alcohol poisoning 58
allergies, anaphylactic shock 91
allergy 90
ambulances, calling 10, 18
amputation 48
anaphylactic shock 91
animal bites 79
ankle injury 67
appendicitis 99
arms
   elbow injury 70
   injuries 70
   slings 106–7, 108
asthma 35
auto-injector 91

B

babies
   changing area safety 114
   choking 28–9
   fever 94
   hypothermia 85
   kitchen safety 112
   resuscitation 19–21
   toys and playthings 117
   unresponsiveness 19–21
back, spine injuries 63
bandages and dressings
   bandages 103

broad-fold bandages 65
   for burns 53
   dressings 102, 104
   embedded objects in wounds 40
   hand bandages 105
   improvised dressings 103
   narrow-fold bandages 65
   roller bandages 105
   sterile pads 104
   triangular bandages 106–7
bathroom safety 116
baths, safety 116
bedroom safety 114–15
beds, safety 115
bee stings 80
berries, poisonous 58
bikes, safety 120
bites
   animal 79
   human 79
   snake 83
   tick 81
bleeding
   abdominal injury 51
   from ear 46
   internal bleeding 49
   nosebleed 45
   scalp wounds 59
   shock 36
   tooth sockets 47
   wounds 38–9
blisters 43
blood sugar levels, diabetic
   emergencies 92
body temperature 15
   fever 94
   heatstroke 89
   hypothermia 84
bones *see* fractures
bottle feeding 112
brachial pulse 15
brain
   concussion 60
   epileptic seizures 97

febrile seizures 96
   meningitis 95
breathing
   anaphylactic shock 91
   asthma 35
   breath holding 32
   chest wounds 50
   choking 28–31
   croup 34
   fume inhalation 33
   hiccups 32
   resuscitating a baby 19–21
   resuscitating a child 17, 22,
   24–5
   spine injuries 63
   strangulation 33
   suffocation 33
   unresponsive baby 19–21
   unresponsive child 22–7
   vital signs 14
broad-fold bandages 65
bruises 74
buggies, safety 121
bunk beds 115
burns 52–7
   chemical burns 55–7
   dressings for 53
   electrical burns 54
   shock after 36

C

calamine lotion 80, 87
carbon monoxide safety 109
cardiopulmonary resuscitation
   see CPR
carpets, safety 111
cars
   car seats 119
   road safety 120
   safety 119
changing areas, safety 114
checking vital signs 14–15
cheekbone injuries 62

chemical burns 55–7
    eye 56
    skin 55
    swallowed chemicals 57
chemicals, garden safety 118
chest
    rib injuries 69
    wounds 50
chest compressions
    resuscitating a baby 20–1
    resuscitating a child 24–5
    spine injuries 63
chip pan fires 11
choking 28–31
circulation
    after bandaging 105
    resuscitation 18
clothing, on fire 11
cold
    frostbite 86
    hypothermia 84–5
cold packs 74, 108
collar bone injury 76
compression, head injuries 60
concussion 60
conforming bandages 103
cookers, safety 113
cots, safety 114
CPR (cardiopulmonary resuscitation)
    babies 20–1
    children 24–5
    spine injuries 63
cramp 73
crossing the road 120
croup 34
crush injury 49
cupboards, safety 113, 116
curtains, safety 111
cuts and grazes 41

D

dehydration
    heat exhaustion 88
    vomiting and diarrhoea 98
diabetic emergencies 92
diarrhoea 98

doors, safety 110, 112
drawers, safety 113
dressings see bandages and dressings
drowning 13
drugs
    poisoning 58
    see also medication
drying machines, safety 113

E

ears
    bleeding from 46
    earache 100
    foreign objects in 77
    wounds 46
elbow injury 70
electricity
    burns 54
    safety 109, 111, 113
    injuries 12
    shock 12, 54
elevation slings 107
embedded objects, in wounds 40
emergencies
    action in 10
    calling an ambulance 10, 18
    choking 28–31
    diabetes 92
    electrical injury 12
    fire 11
    seizures 96–7
    unresponsiveness 14–29
    water incident 13
epileptic seizures 97
eyes
    chemical burns 56
    foreign objects in 76
    wounds 44

F

face
    cheekbone injuries 62
    jaw injuries 62
    mouth wounds 47
    nose injuries 62

fainting 93
febrile seizures 96
feet
    blisters 43
    cramp 73
    frostbite 86
    injuries 64
fever 94
    febrile seizures 96
fingers
    amputation 48
    frostbite 86
    trapped fingers 71
fire 11
    chip pan fires 11
    clothing on fire 11
    escaping from 11
    home safety 109
fire blankets 112
fire extinguishers 112
fireplaces, safety 111
first aid kit 102–3
    household items 108
fits see seizures
flannels 108
floors, safety 110, 112
food poisoning 113
foot see feet
foreign objects
    in ear 77
    in eye 76
    in nose 78
    swallowed 78
    in wounds 40
fractures
    ankle 67
    arm 70
    collar bone 68
    foot 66
    hand 71
    jaw 62
    leg 64–5
    pelvis 64
    ribs 69
    skull 61
    spine 63
fridges, safety 113

frostbite 86
fume inhalation 33
furniture, safety 111

G

garages, safety 119
gardens, safety 118
gas
    inhalation 33
    safety 109
gauze swabs 102
grazes 41

H

halls, safety 110
hands
    amputated fingers 48
    bandages 105
    frostbite 86
    hand injuries 71
    trapped fingers 71
head
    cheekbone injuries 62
    head injuries 60–1
    jaw injuries 62
    mouth wounds 47
    nose injuries 62
    scalp wounds 59
    skull fractures 61
heart massage
    babies 20–1
    children 24–5
heat exhaustion 88
heat rash 87
heaters, safety 111
heatstroke 89
hiccups 32
high-voltage current 12
highchairs, safety 112
hobs, safety 113
home safety 109–19
hornet stings 86
human bites 79
hypoallergenic tape 102
hypothermia 84–5

I

immunisations
    foreign travel 122
    tetanus 42
improvised dressings 103
improvised slings 106
infected wounds 42
inhalation, fumes 33
injections, Epipen 91
insects
    in ear 77
    insect repellent 122
    stings 80
internal bleeding 49

J

jaw injuries 62
jellyfish stings 82
joints
    ankle injury 67
    elbow injury 70
    knee injury 66

K

kitchen film, as emergency
    dressing 108
kitchens, safety 112–13
knee injury 66

L

legs
    ankle injury 67
    cramp 73
    injuries 64–5
    knee injury 66
    splints 65
limbs, amputation 48

M

marine puncture wound 82
medication
    asthma 35

drug poisoning 58
    Epipen 91
meningitis 95
mouth
    bleeding from tooth socket
        47
    burns 52
    toothache 101
    wounds 47
muscles, cramp 73

N

narrow-fold bandages 65
nettle rash 80
nose
    foreign objects in 78
    injuries 62
    nosebleeds 45

O

ovens, safety 113

P

paediatric AED 23
pelvic injury 64
pillow cases, as emergency
    dressings 108
plants, poisonous 58, 118
plasters 102
plastic bags, emergency
    dressings 108
play, safety 112, 117
playgrounds, safety 121
poisoning
    drug 58
    alcohol 58
    plants 58, 118
prams, safety 121
pressure-change earache
    100
pulse
    brachial 15
    checking 15
    radial 15

R

radial pulse 15
rashes
  heat rash 58
  meningitis 95
  nettle rash 80
recovery position
  babies 21
  children 26–7
rescue breathing
  after drowning 13
  resuscitating a baby 19–21
  resuscitating a child 23–5
rib injuries 69
road safety 120
roller bandages 102, 105

S

safety in the home 109–19
  bathrooms 116
  bedrooms 114–15
  electricity 109
  fire 109
  garage and car safety 119
  gardens 118
  gas 109
  hall and stairs 110
  kitchens 112–13
  sitting rooms 111
  toys and playthings 117
safety pins 103
scalds 52–3
scalp wounds 59
scissors 102
seizures
  epileptic 97
  febrile 96
severe bleeding 38
sheds, safety 118
sheets, as emergency dressings 108
shock 36–7
  anaphylactic 91
  electrical 12
showers, safety 116
sitting rooms, safety 111

skin
  chemical burns 55
  heat rash 87
  meningitis rash 95
  nettle rash 80
  sun protection 122
  sunburn 87
skull fracture 61
slings 70, 106–7
  collar bone injury 68
  elevation slings 107
  hand injuries 71
  improvised slings 106
smoke detectors 109
smoke inhalation 33
snake bites 83
spinal injuries 63
splinters 75
splints, leg 65
sprains, ankle 67
stairs, safety 110
sterile dressings 102, 104
stings
  insect 80
  jellyfish 82
  weever fish 82
stomachache 99
strangers, talking to 121
strangulation 33
street safety 120
suffocation 33
sun protection 122
sunburn 87
swallowed chemicals 57
swallowed foreign objects 78
swellings 74

T

tables, safety 113
tape, hypoallergenic 102
teeth
  bleeding from tooth socket 47
  toothache 101
telephones, in an emergency 10
temperature 15
  fever 94

heat exhaustion 88
heat rash 87
heatstroke 89
hypothermia 84–5
sunburn 87
tetanus 41, 42
throat, burns 52
tick bites 81
toes, frostbite 86
toilets, safety 116
tooth sockets, bleeding from 47
toothache 101
toys, safety 115, 117
trapped fingers 71
travel 122
triangular bandages 106–7
tweezers 102

U

unresponsiveness 15, 16–27
  AED 23
  anaphylactic shock 91
  babies 19–21
  calling an ambulance 18
  children 22–5
  choking 29, 31
  diabetic emergencies 92
  epileptic seizures 97
  fainting 93
  febrile seizures 96
  head injuries 60–1
  recovery position 26–7

V

vaccinations
  foreign travel 122
  tetanus 41, 42
vital signs, checking 14–15
vomiting 98

W

washing machines, safety 113
wasp stings 80
wastebins, safety 112

water
  drowning 13
  incident 13
  safety 118
weever fish stings 82
windows, safety 115
work surfaces, safety 113
wounds
  abdominal 51

amputation 48
animal bites 79
bleeding 38–9
blisters 43
chest 50
crush injury 49
cuts and grazes 41
ear 46
embedded objects in 40

eye 44
infected 42
marine 82
mouth 47
scalp 59
splinters 75

Acknowledgments

Dorling Kindersley would like to thank Phil Gamble, Sachin Singh, and Anjali Sachar for the illustrations; and Suefa Lee for editorial assisstance and indexing.

The publisher would like to thank the following for their kind permission to reproduce their photographs:
(Key: a-above; b-below/bottom; c-centre; f-far; l-left; r-right; t-top)
21 Lloyd Sturdy: British Red Cross br; **81** Wikipedia: CDC/ James Gathany br
All other images © Dorling Kindersley
For further information see: **www.dkimages.com**
Dorling Kindersley would like to thank:
Joe Mulligan, Head of First Aid Education, Nadine Threader, Jane Keogh, and Andrew Farrar from the British Red Cross; Cardiac Science for the loan of the paediatric AED; Hilary Bird for the index; the following for modelling:
Children Aleena Awan, Navaz Awan, Max Buckingham, Madeline Cameron, Alfie Clarke, Amy Davies, Thomas Davies, James Dow, Kyla Edwards, Austin Enil, Lia Foa, Maya Foa, Jessica Forge, Kashi Gorton, Emily Gorton, Thomas Greene, Alexander Harrison, Rupert Harrison, Ben Harrison, Jessica Harris-Voss, Hannah Headam, Jake Hutton, Rosemary Kaloki, Winnie Kaloki, Ella Kaye, Maddy Kaye, Jade Lamb, Emily Leney, Harriet Lord, Daniel Lord, Crispin Lord, Ailsa McCaughrean, Fiona Maine, Tom Maine, Kincaid Malik-White, Maija Marsh, Oliver Metcalf, Eloise Morgan, Tom Razazan, Jimmy Razazan, Georgia Ritter, Rebecca Sharples, Ben Sharples, Thomas Sharples, Ben Walker, Robyn Walker, Amy Beth Walton Evans, Hanna Warren-Green, Simon Weekes, Joseph Weir, Lily Ziegler.
Adults Shaila Awan, Claire le Bas, Joanna Benwell, Angela Cameron, Georgina Davies, Marion Davies, Sophie Dow, Tina Edwards, Rachel Fitchett, Emma Foa, Emma Forge, Caroline Greene, Susan Harrison, Victoria Harrison, Julia Harris-Voss, Roy Headam, Emma Hutton, Helga Lien Evans, Sylvie Jordan, Jane Kaloki, David Kaye, Louise Kaye, Philip Lord, Geraldine McCaughrean, Diana Maine, Brian Marsh, Jonathan Metcalf, Francoise Morgan, Juliette Norsworthy, Anna Pizzi, Hossein Razazan, Angela Sharples, John Sharples, Nadine Threader, Miranda Tunbridge, Vanessa Walker, Catherine Warren-Green, Toni Weekes, Robert Ziegler.
Make-up: Wendy Holmes, Pebbles, Geoff Portas.
Additional photography Andy Crawford, Steve Gorton, Ray Mollers, Suzannah Price, Dave Rudkin, Steve Shott, Lloyd Sturdy.

Useful telephone numbers

IN AN EMERGENCY DIAL 999 or 112. ASK FOR THE AMBULANCE (medical emergencies only), FIRE BRIGADE, OR POLICE

FOR MEDICAL ADVICE
IN ENGLAND, SCOTLAND AND N.IRELAND: 111
IN WALES: 0845 4647

Doctor
Name: _____
Address: _____
Telephone: _____
Out of hours telephone: _____
Surgery Hours: _____

Health Visitor
Name: _____
Clinic Address: _____
_____
Telephone: _____
Clinic Hours: _____

Dentist
Name: _____
Address: _____
Telephone: _____
Out of hours telephone: _____
Surgery Hours: _____

Hospital Accident & Emergency
Address: _____
_____
Telephone: _____

Late Night Chemist
Address: _____
Telephone: _____

Local Police
Telephone: _____

Gas Emergency Service
Telephone: _____

Electricity Emergency Service
Telephone: _____

Water Emergency Service
Telephone: _____

Notes
_____
_____
_____
_____
_____
_____
_____
_____
_____
_____
_____
_____